Vulnerability, Churches, and HIV

Vulnerability, Churches, and HIV

Edited by
GÖRAN GUNNER

☙PICKWICK *Publications* • Eugene, Oregon

VULNERABILITY, CHURCHES, AND HIV

Church of Sweden, Research Series 1

Copyright © 2009 Trossamfundet Svenska kyrkan (Church of Sweden). All rights reserved. Except for brief quotations in critical publications or reviews, no part of this book may be reproduced in any manner without prior written permission from the publisher. Write: Permissions, Wipf and Stock, 199 W. 8th Ave., Suite 3, Eugene, OR 97401.

Pickwick Publications
A Division of Wipf and Stock Publishers
199 West 8th Avenue, Suite 3
Eugene, Oregon 97401

www.wipfandstock.com

ISBN 13: 978-1-60608-058-0

Scripture quotations are from the New Revised Standard Version Bible © 1989, Division of Christian Education of the National Council of the Churches of Christ in the United States of America. Used by permission. All rights reserved.

Manufactured in the U.S.A.

Contents

Contributors vii

Introduction: Vulnerability, Churches, and HIV—*Göran Gunner* 1

1. On Being an HIV-positive Church and Doing Theology in an HIV-positive World—*Musa W. Dube* 5
2. The Body of Christ Has HIV—*Susanne Rappmann* 24
3. Jesus, the Leper, and HIV and AIDS: Suffering, Solidarity, and Structural Transformation—*Kenneth R. Overberg, S.J.* 33
4. Women and the Choices They Hold: Hope in the HIV Epidemic—*Edwina Ward* 52
5. A Pastoral Letter from the Bishops of the Church of Sweden about HIV from a Global Perspective 68

Resources 95

Bibliography 99

Contributors

Prof. Musa W. Dube is Professor of New Testament at Botswana university, Gaborone.

Dr. Göran Gunner is Associate Professor at the University of Uppsala and works as a Researcher at Church of Sweden Research Department.

Prof. Kenneth R. Overberg, S.J., is Professor at the Theology Graduate Program, Xavier University, Cincinnati, USA.

Dr. Susanne Rappmann got her degree from the Department of Religious Studies and Theology, Karlstad University and is working as a parish priest in Sweden.

Dr. Edwina Ward is working at the School of Religion and Theology at the University of KwaZulu-Natal, South Africa.

Archbishop Anders Wejryd is Archbishop of Church of Sweden.

Introduction

Vulnerability, Churches, and HIV

Göran Gunner

THE HIV[1] PANDEMIC POSES serious challenges to the church and to theology. The global society has been transformed by the impact of HIV and AIDS[2]. Calculations by UNAIDS indicate almost 33.2 million HIV-infected[3]. The loss of lives through HIV and AIDS is one tragic consequence of the disease. In addition, the pandemic has caused enormous human suffering to individuals, and has also affected families and entire societies. The health and social challenges following in the wake of the disease have become major obstacles to organizing and maintaining sustainable societies and global justice.

In this context, the church—on the local, national, and international levels—needs to listen, learn and, not the least, to respond in order to form a solid basis for its own actions and its future.

> The church cannot be a credible witness in the context of HIV/AIDS unless it understands the nature of change in people's lives, the factors that contribute to them, as well as their fears and hopes, and is willing to change itself to become a more loving, inclusive community for all God's people.[4]

The presence of HIV and AIDS in society and in the church requires the church to become an HIV- and AIDS-competent church. This book is one of several measures intended to challenge the Church of Sweden to become more HIV- and AIDS-competent.

1. Human Immunodeficiency Virus.
2. Acquired Immunodeficiency Syndrome.
3. "2007 AIDS epidemic update."
4. "Facing AIDS."

The bishops of the Church of Sweden have addressed the question of HIV in a special statement, *A pastoral letter from the bishops of the Church of Sweden concerning HIV in a global perspective*, with a preface by Archbishop Anders Wejryd. After presenting their views on the HIV situation, and elaborating theological and ethical aspects of HIV, the bishops offer recommendations for both the national and the international arenas. The recommendations are addressed to among others Swedish decision-making bodies, international organizations, patent-holders and decision-makers in the pharmaceutical industry and, not least, to church parishes, employees and leaders.

With the pastoral letter, the bishops join theologians around the world who are working actively to interpret the roles of the Gospel, the church, and society in the face of the HIV-pandemic. To note just a few examples of books on the subject that have been published during the past few years: *Grant Me Justice!* edited by Musa W. Dube and Musimbi Kanyoro; Donald Messer's *Breaking the Conspiracy of Silence: Christian Churches and the Global AIDS Crisis*; Maria Cimperman's *When God's People Have HIV/AIDS*; Kenneth R. Overberg's *Ethics and AIDS*; and two recent books by Ezra Chitando, *Living with Hope* and *Acting in Hope*.

Every two years, the Church of Sweden's Research Department invites the academic society to give inputs from their research work. As part of "Days for Researchers 2007," some of the above-mentioned authors and some others, all representing different geographical locations, were invited to participate.

Professor Musa W. Dube from the University of Botswana in Gaborone, Botswana, delivered a key-note address, "On Being an HIV-Positive Church & Doing Theology in an HIV-Positive World." Other participants included: Professor Kenneth R. Overberg, S.J. from Xavier University, in Cincinnati, USA; Dr. Edwina Ward from the University of KwaZulu-Natal, South Africa; and Dr. Susanne Rappmann, a parish priest in Sweden.

All of them participated in seminars entitled "The Vulnerable, Churches and HIV" and "Churches infected and affected by HIV"; their contributions are included in this volume. The authors address HIV and AIDS as a reality within the churches, and as a challenge for theology and churches. They discuss HIV as creating vulnerability and stigmatization, but also how it is related to such problems as structural injustice, poverty,

Introduction: Vulnerability, Churches, and HIV

gender inequality, sexual harassment, and discrimination based on gender or sexual orientation.

In addition, the authors discuss alternatives relating to healthy and safe sexuality, human relationships, and the church as a caring and healing community. The authors also show that it is important for the church to become a story-telling and story-sharing community, as well as a Bible-reading and -interpreting community.

Some other initiatives of the Church of Sweden should also be mentioned. The Central Church Office has established a special desk officer to serve as "Policy Advisor on hiv and aids."

In 2005, together with partners in Africa, the Church of Sweden initiated a master's degree program entitled, "Theological Project for of HIV/AIDS." The overall goals and objectives were stated as:

- enabling the African churches to take a proactive role in civil society
- promoting action programmes to deal with the consequences of the HIV/ AIDS pandemic
- encouraging theological reflection through the action-reflection model, according to which theological students are trained to serve their communities.

Participating in the master's program have been 36 students from four institutions in Africa: Stellenbosch University and KwaZulu-Natal University in South Africa, Makumira University College in Tanzania, and Ethiopian Graduate School of Theology. Each institution was invited to select ten students for one academic year of research and study at the master's level.

A central issue addressed by the project has been how the church lives, celebrates and does theology in the midst of an ongoing HIV and AIDS pandemic. Specific questions have included: How to speak about God in this situation? What is the role of the church and religion in the work of stopping the spread of the HIV pandemic? What special concerns and problems are raised? In what ways are cultural and gender diversity manifested? In what ways are theological reflection and local experience contributing to theological studies and church activities? The resulting master's theses are currently being prepared for publication.[5]

---

5. Ward, *A Theology of HIV*.

Vulnerability, Churches, and HIV

With these introductory remarks, I invite you to read *Vulnerability, Churches, and HIV*, starting with the contributions of the researchers, followed by the pastoral letter from the bishops of the Church of Sweden.

1

On Being an HIV-positive Church and Doing Theology in an HIV-positive World

Musa W. Dube

An HIV+ Church
Is an embodied Church
It is a Church living with AIDS
It is a compassionate community
It is an active and activist Church
It is a story-telling Church
A listening Church
A lamenting Church
A prophetic Church
A gender-sensitive Church
An orphaned-child sensitive Church
A People Living with HIV and AIDS Sensitive Church
A justice-birthing and -embracing Church
A Christological Church
Living in the resurrection power
The power of Christ
Who is HIV+[1]

The starting point in this mission and ministry is admitting that ultimately we are all HIV positive. As long as we deny our own vulnerability and risk, rebuff our own oneness with the suffering of the world, and pretend we are separate from our infected and affected sisters and brothers, then perhaps we best step aside

---

1. Cf. Russell-Coons, "We have AIDS," 39.

Vulnerability, Churches, and HIV

(. . .) Turn the page only if you can honestly say, we are all HIV positive.[2]

THERE IS A CONDOM IN THE CHURCH!

In the second half of the 1980's when we were beginning to hear about HIV, a girlfriend brought me a condom. She said to me, *Nnaaka tsaya condom e. Ke malatsi a mogare. Fa go ka diragala gore o be onale mongwe, oitshereletse,* that is:

> My young sister, take this condom. If it happens that you get sexually involved do not be found unprepared, these are the days of HIV. Protect yourself.

Feeling quite skeptical about such an event happening to me, given that I was a subscriber to premarital abstinence to sex, I nonetheless accepted the condom. I put it in my purse and I forgot about it for a long time.

One morning I went to church and sat next to a woman with a child. I was holding my purse and the child immediately reached for it. I let the child have it. The child sat down and began to pull out everything in my purse. I was quite relaxed watching the child dismantle the contents of my purse. Suddenly, I remembered: the condom in my purse! As you can imagine, I jumped and retrieved my purse from the child.

I was virtually shaking. "What if the child had pulled the condom out? How would I explain to my church that I carry a condom in my purse?" As soon as the service ended, I found the nearest rubbish bin and disposed the condom, thanking the heavens that I remembered before I got stigmatized for sexual immorality; for if AIDS was there, what did the church and its members have to do with it?

THERE IS NO DENYING: HIV AND AIDS ARE IN THE CHURCH

But that was about twenty-two years ago. We have come a long way in the past twenty-six years of living with HIV and AIDS in our world. The question of whether or not the church and its members have anything to do with HIV and AIDS is no longer debatable. It is obvious. There is no denying: that HIV and AIDS are in the church.

---

2. Messer, *Breaking the Conspiracy*, 38.

For example, in the first half of this year, I was running workshops for pastors on mainstreaming HIV and AIDS in worship in Botswana. I was training them on how to use *Africa Praying: A Handbook on HIV/AIDS Sensitive Sermons and Liturgy*. On the second day of these training workshops, I usually employ a healing and memorial service, whose aim is to break the stigma and heal the participants.[3] The liturgy used involves coming forward to light a candle for a relative, friend, workmate, neighbor or church mate who has been infected or affected by HIV and AIDS.

When I first designed the service order back in 2003, it was meant to assist church people to realize that HIV and AIDS is not just "out there," affecting only non-Christians and the so called sinners; rather, that we are all affected by HIV and AIDS. And indeed, as a church, we are also infected by HIV and AIDS; for if one member is infected, we are all infected (1 Cor 12:26a).

The theological framework of a church that identifies itself with the affected and People Living with HIV and AIDS (PLWHA) was critical in breaking the silence and building a compassionate and healing church in the HIV and AIDS context.

In the early days of employing the service, when there was still a lot of denial, many people would come forward and light a candle for general identities such as "all orphans, all people living with HIV and AIDS, all widows, all caregivers or the sick that my church visits in the hospital." Very few people openly said I light this candle for my child, my spouse, my sibling, my HIV and AIDS status. The trend was to generalize and to distance oneself. But the few who would come out and say that I am admitting for the first time that my parent, sibling, relative, spouse, or friend died of AIDS constituted great strides in the struggle against HIV and AIDS. They assisted us in breaking the silence and stigma, but above all in highlighting the obvious—namely that we are an HIV-positive church.

Early this year, when I ran training workshops for church ministers in Botswana, there was a marked difference towards this worship service. Each worshiper took time to light not just one candle, but several candles for their children who died, for the orphans that they are raising, for parents who died, for siblings, for fiancées, for friends and relatives who are living with HIV and AIDS, some being cared for and others being

---

3. Dube, *Africa Praying*, 43–45.

on antiretroviral therapy (ARV). Indeed, there were some who identified themselves as PLWHA.

In one such workshop, where we had twenty-five participants, the service went on for two hours, since people wanted to tell the stories surrounding their relatives and friends and how they have been affected and infected by HIV and AIDS. I sat back and let the storytelling process take its full course, since for many it was the very first time that they had an opportunity in the worship space to tell their stories of living in an HIV-positive world and how they have been directly affected.

Of course, there was lot of crying since some were admitting for the first time that their relatives died of AIDS. I remember two sisters who had lost their mother to AIDS. The eldest discovered it in the death certificate, which she hid from all her other siblings. The other siblings found the certificate, read it and kept the secret to themselves. Consequently, they had never talked about it or admitted to another that they knew it until they discovered their shared knowledge through the service.

I remember a pastor from an evangelical church who stood up and said, "My father and my brother died of AIDS."

In sum, the response in 2007 was overwhelmingly positive compared with 2003 when I started using the service order. In fact, I have now found myself struggling with ethical questions of caring for those who really began to cry, and the ethical responsibility of inviting people to divulge information that caused them pain, without ensuring that there will be continued counseling. While the service began to raise ethical questions (which I believe can be addressed by providing counseling services) I remember one of the participants saying:

> If a church minister can rise and speaking publicly, as I have seen them here saying, "I lost three children to AIDS, and I am busy caring for their offspring," then we have come a long way and we have hope that HIV and AIDS stigma can be laid to rest.

For the purposes of this discussion, these services confirm the obvious—namely, that the church is HIV+, the church has AIDS. This statement is not only ecclesiological and factually correct, it is also Christological correct. I will now briefly highlight the relevant concepts, below.

AN EMBODIED CHURCH: LIVING IN AND THROUGH THE HIV AND AIDS EPIDEMIC

We are very much an embodied church that lives in the physical matter of our bodies and in the world. Indeed we need to remind ourselves that in the Johannine farewell discourse, Jesus prayed that they should not be taken out of this world—but to remain in it (John 17:13–16). It is factually correct to say the church is HIV+ and living with AIDS, for the church consists of those amongst us who are physically and emotionally living with HIV and AIDS. They include those amongst us who have the HI virus in their physical bodies, those who are affected either through caring for the orphaned, the sick, and the widowed, and through grief in the loss of relatives, friends, and the loss of hope for the future.

We are concretely affected and infected because we have come to live on the edge, on uncertainty about the future. It is also factually correct to say the church is HIV+, for the church lives in a world that is HIV+. More than 60 million of our members around the world have been infected by HIV and more than a third of these have died—and we, the church, are in this HIV+ world. Accordingly, there is no need for any special pleading on this matter: We are an HIV+ world and church in every way that this disease has manifested itself.

But to say that the church is concretely HIV+ essentially means that the church, like an HIV+ body, has lived and manifested all the stages of the virus in more ways than one, just like a physical body that is infected. As an HIV+ church, we have gone through a hidden period of incubation, when we hoped that the virus is "out there"—attacking anyone else but us. During that time, we let the virus entrench itself in our bodies, eating away our immunity.

The depletion of our immunity as communities of faith became clear through some stigmatizing attitudes that characterized some of our voices. We began to gradually notice that we were infected when we manifested fear, indifference, denial, and when some of our members became sick, when some died, when we buried some, and when we had to provide grief counseling to our surviving members and ourselves.

Yet we continued with the denial, characterizing our PLWHA-members as exceptions—and indeed, in some quarters, as sinners. Our denial was clear in the lack of a theology of compassion, healing, hope, prophecy, and resurrection. We still prayed and hoped that the epidemic would pass us by, and that we would assist those who are living and dying of HIV and AIDS "out there."

But it was not at all out there. It was right in our physical bodies and in our body, the church. Opportunistic infections began to show more visibly on our physical bodies, and we had to counsel ourselves that it was not out there; it was *right here*. The epidemic was in the church, as it is in the world.

By this time in some parts of the world, our pastors were spending too much time visiting the sick, counseling grieved orphans/widows, and too much time burying. Every burial, the total of which quickly expanded the boundaries of the graveyard, was a concrete reminder to the church that we are not immune to HIV.

It was when death was becoming a daily bread in many churches that we began to accept that we are a church living with HIV and AIDS. It was then that we began to seek our own healing and to be healers for one another in the church and in the larger community. It was then that we began to proclaim life in the light of invasion by AIDS-death. It was then that we began to proclaim hope in the face of ghastly hopelessness. It was then that we begin to proclaim healing in the face of opportunistic infections that characterized the body of Christ. It was then that we sought to be a compassionate community.

I have to say that I wish the story of an HIV+ church had unfolded in this simple linear fashion. If that were the case, this moment of time would for me be a moment of celebration, a time when I could say that the church is now an HIV- and AIDS-competent church that does not respond with, silence, denial, indifference, stigmatization, injustice, hopelessness, death, and incurability.

If the story had unfolded in that way, I would now at least be saying that the church now tests for the disease, knows its status, employs all effective means to prevent new infections, practices compassion, assumes a clear prophetic role, and takes its treatment faithfully and consistently. I would be saying that the church is now a realm of compassion, hope, healing, life, resurrection, and prophecy. I would be saying that the church, worldwide, is now a formidable and effective army of healing in the struggle against HIV and AIDS.

The story of the church and HIV and AIDS has, however, been anything but simple. It has been characterized by multiple parallel plots, some of which include flash-backs, many of which ended in failure, i.e. plots that never developed. The latter are evident in many infantilized churches that remain steeped in silence, denial, indifference, and stigmatization.

Churches in this category still say it is out there, but not here. They do not plan and budget for curbing the spread of HIV and AIDS and advocating affordable quality care. Such infantilized churches have not yet developed a theology that enables its members to be an effective army in the struggle against HIV and AIDS. Such churches do not have policies that must guide all its members on a systematic and effective response to the global HIV and AIDS crisis.

Indeed, infantilized churches do not raise their voices against the structural forces that generate and maintain poverty and gender inequality. They have no prophecy for this injustice-driven epidemic. These underdeveloped churches in the HIV and AIDS drama remain oblivious to the fact that we have 15 million orphaned children, a total of 40 million HIV+ members of our world. They remain unmoved by the fact that we are a world that has lost about 25 million people in just about twenty five years of the epidemic.

I am sure you will agree with me that, in every country, our church historians and sociologists have a lot of work ahead of them to document the story of how the churches responded to the HI viruses that attacked our congregations, communities, countries and continents. That work will include telling the story of churches that managed to respond,—how they responded, and how they played or failed to play their parts. Church historians have a job ahead of them to highlight for us the best practices that developed in the church family, as a way of motivating other churches by providing clear and helpful models.

A COMPASSIONATE CHURCH: IF ONE MEMBER SUFFERS, WE ALL SUFFER

But let me return to the idea that it is ecclesiological and theologically correct to say that the church is HIV+. For, the church is the body of Christ—and if one member suffers, we all suffer with them (1 Cor 12:26). The fact that the church cannot distance itself from the suffering of its members implies two things: First, the church is a compassionate body. Second, the church always exists in relation to all its members and to all humanity; it is communal in nature.

Given these two aspects, the church is by theological definition a compassionate community that cannot—I mean should not—distance itself from the suffering of its members—if it is a church. This does not necessarily depend on one's geographical location or one's HIV status. Rather, there are two significant issues: first, realizing that we are all members of God's creation; second, realizing that belonging to the community of believers that call themselves a church carries with it certain obligations. In the theological thinking of church, the earth and everything in it belongs to the Lord; and further, if one member suffers, we all suffer.

The church, in other words, should be fundamentally a compassionate community, one that identifies with rather than distances itself from its marginalized and suffering members, wherever they are located. To say that the church is HIV-positive, to say that the church has AIDS, is to say that it is a compassionate community. Compassion is therefore central to the identity of being a church community. Accordingly, J. P. Heath asserts that "God has allowed HIV to heal the church, to force us to become Christian."[4]

In their book, *Compassion: A Reflection on the Christian Life*, Henri J. M. Nouwen, Donald P. Mc Neill, and Douglas A. Morrison hold that:

> Compassion asks us to go where it hurts, to enter into places of pain, to share in brokenness, fear, confusion, and anguish. Compassion challenges us to cry out with those in misery, to mourn with those who are lonely, to weep with those in tears. Compassion requires us to be weak with the weak, vulnerable with the vulnerable, and powerless with the powerless. Compassion means full immersion in the condition of being human.[5]

Sally Purvis' definition of compassion is a useful addition to the above:

> (. . .) not only *the capacity to be moved by pain* (. . .) *of another;* compassion also denotes *an important source of energy we need to respond*—to right a wrong when we can; to protest when we are impotent to effect change; and to support the conditions for flourishing that we observe. Compassion, in this view, is a robust concept that includes *not only motivation but movement* (emphasis added).[6]

---

4. Heath, "HIV- and AIDS," 31.
5. Nouwen et al., *Compassion*, 4.
6. Purvis, "Compassion," 52.

Indeed, the above definitions indicate that compassion is an active verb. If compassion means to suffer with, to enter into places of pain, to go where it hurts, to share in brokenness, fear, confusion and anguish, then a compassionate church is not a passive community. A compassionate church is an active church. In the HIV and AIDS era, where we are ever so tempted to isolate the PLWHA, acknowledging that the church is a compassionate community means that, we cannot afford to be indifferent, to be silent, or to stigmatize. We cannot afford to not have an agenda in the struggle against HIV and AIDS. It is simply out of character.

Acknowledging that we are a Church Living with HIV and AIDS means that we are a community that has the energy and the strength needed to be in solidarity with those amongst us who are PLWHA and others who are affected. We are inseparable. Acknowledging that we are an HIV-positive church denotes our engagement, involvement and activity in the struggle against HIV and AIDS rather than indifference, silence, stigmatization and discrimination. We are a church living with HIV and AIDS—Children Living with HIV and AIDS (CLWHA).

Being an HIV+ church thus means we are active in the search for and implementation of HIV and AIDS prevention. We bear in our own bodies the wounds of AIDS. Being an HIV+ church means that we are active in searching for and providing quality care with and for PLWHA, the orphaned, the widowed, the discriminated, and the disempowered. Being an HIV+ church means that the struggle against HIV and AIDS is not peripheral to our business, rather it is central to our worship, to our articulation of Christian faith.

An HIV+ church is therefore not merely assisting the government or non-governmental organizations (NGOs), or PLWHA, or the affected groups such as orphans, widows, and the sick. Rather, an HIV+ church is actively involved in the struggle against HIV and AIDS because it is an inherent characteristic and role of a church—to be a compassionate community. It is at the core of the church to be compassionate, to be a church that is on the move and moved by compassion.

I want to go back to the above description of the churches of Botswana and explore three aspects of being a storytelling, lamenting, and prophetic church, as central to being an HIV+ church. I will conclude by exploring the notion of a HIV+ church as a Christological correct posture.

Vulnerability, Churches, and HIV

A STORYTELLING CHURCH

Why should storytelling characterize an HIV+ positive church? Storytelling allows us to hear "the Other"—those amongst us who are affected and living with HIV and AIDS. First, storytelling calls us to become listening communities. It calls us to be present for the most marginalized and oppressed. Storytelling calls us into hearing each other. It creates a safe space for being vulnerable. In so doing it provides a birth space for the becoming of compassionate communities. When we listen to a story, we are invited into the world of the story and the storyteller, and hence called to take our part within their story. Storytelling bears the fruits of empathy, solidarity, networking, and collaboration.

Since the storytellers in the context of HIV and AIDS are those amongst us who are affected and living with HIV, a storytelling space becomes an essential instrument by which compassion occurs. Storytelling space becomes the space where the church is transformed to become a compassionate community. Without listening, without allowing ourselves to hear, without allowing ourselves to identify with the stories of "the Other," we deny ourselves the transformative power of becoming a compassionate community.

The gist of being a storytelling church and a listening church is to create a space for birthing a compassionate community. In this space, those amongst us who are PLWHA and others who are affected become central agents in the formation and giving of compassion.[7] Their voices, stories and lived experience become the foundation of a theology of compassion. Compassion, in other words, does not patronize, silence or replace PLWHA and the affected as active subjects in the struggle against HIV and AIDS. Rather, compassion empowers companionship and solidarity. A theology of compassion is a theology of empowerment and liberation that fully recognizes the human dignity and initiative of the oppressed and marginalized in working out their own salvation and inviting us to realize that our salvation is inseparably tied to their salvation.

Consequently, storytelling is emerging as a central method for highlighting the situation of women and the girl-child in the HIV and AIDS struggle, and for articulating a feminist/womanist HIV and AIDS theology of healing and liberation. Commenting on the storytelling method, Isabel Apawo Phiri and Sarojini Nadar note that:

---

7. Heath, "HIV- and AIDS," 27–31.

African women theologians have frequently and unabashedly used this method of theologizing as a powerful and potent method to critique oppressive practices in African Religion-culture.[8]

According to Ackermann, "telling stories is intrinsic to claiming one's identity and in the process finding impulses for hope."[9] In terms of research, the storytelling method lands itself well to both field and library-based HIV and AIDS research. Elisinah Chauke's article represents a great example of using data to collect fieldwork data.[10]

Storytelling also provides a powerful space of healing. In the HIV-positive world that is characterized by silence, stigma and discrimination, we are sicker than we realize. As J. P. Heath points out, "It's not only people living with HIV who need healing, but also the church."[11] In the storytelling space, we divine and diagnose ourselves, since first and foremost we break the silence and speak out our fears, hopelessness and loss of a secured future. In sharing stories, we open the hidden wounds of how HIV has not only attacked our physical bodies, but has also invaded our spirits, souls, emotions, and communities.

In sharing stories those amongst us who are PLWHA articulate their experiences, their encounter with stigma and discrimination, their fears of the future, their hopes, and hopelessness. But in sharing these stories we come upon another horizon, where the rising sun bears healing on its wings to us.[12] This healing occurs precisely because, in storytelling, we birth compassionate communities that are a formidable force of hope and healing. As compassionate communities are birthed, we discover that we are not alone; that together we are much stronger than the HI virus. In compassionate communities we discover life and hope for the future, rather than the shadow of death. Birthing compassionate communities empowers all of us and heals us. It is on these grounds that I have elsewhere argued that, when:

---

8. Phiri and Nadar, "Introduction," 8. Examples here include: Chauke, "Theological Challenges," 128–48; Ackermann, "Tamar's Cry," 27–59; Ackermann, "HIV- and AIDS," 221–42; Moyo, "Navigating," 243–57; Landman, "Spiritual," 189–208; Dube, "Twenty-Two Years," 186–200.

9. Ackermann, "Tamar's Cry," 41.

10. Chauke, "Theological Challenges," 128–48.

11. Heath, "HIV- and AIDS," 31.

12. Ackermann, "HIV- and AIDS," 48.

(...) we listen to each other's stories, we create a space of breaking the silences, of understanding, of empathy, of being prophetic to one another and hopefully of giving justice a better deal.[13]

Story-telling, therefore not only gives birth to compassionate churches, it also facilitates lamenting and prophetic churches, two aspects that I wish to highlight as defining characteristics of an HIV+ church.

A LAMENTING CHURCH

In the above description of Botswana churches, I also mentioned tears—the tears of an HIV-positive church. An HIV-positive church is a lamenting church. The fact that the HIV and AIDS crisis entails long suffering, stigma, discrimination, injustice, death and, more often than not, loss of the future, lamentation is inevitable.[14]

But what is lament? According to Denise Ackermann it is important to note that a theology of lament is not the same as a theology of hopelessness and victimization.[15] Rather, lamentation is a framework that insists on exposing injustice and calling for justice to be established. Those who lament are making a social protest against the oppressive conditions of their existence as unacceptable; they are underlining the need for transformation. Their voices are insisting on the need to let justice roll down into our streets and homes. Lamentations are in themselves a call for the establishment of justice.

For theologians, the hermeneutic of lament and its theology is quite central. Consequently, when one turns to the works of the Circle of African Women Theologians, who have been focusing on HIV and AIDS for the past five years, the tears of African women theologians are both loud and silent.[16] Like Rachel, Circle women's voices are heard, "wailing and loud lamentation, Rachel weeping for her children; she refused to be consoled" (Matt 2:18). The lamenting voices of Circle women are heard, calling for the dismantling of patriarchy, which in the HIV and AIDS context has become a death-sanction to women through its feminization of poverty, violence against women, and the disempowerment of women

---

13. Dube, *HIV/AIDS*, 109.

14. Ackermann, "Tamar's Cry," 27–59; Boniface-Male, "Allow Me," 169–85; Kanyoro "Preface: Breaking," xi–xii.

15. Ackermann, "HIV- and AIDS," 49.

16. Ackermann, "Tamar's Cry"; Boniface-Male, "Allow Me."

from the ability to make choices over their lives and bodies. It follows that a theology of lamentation points to the fact that an HIV+ church must be a prophetic community, a point I wish to address.

A PROPHETIC CHURCH

We have now had twenty-six years of living with HIV in our world. During this time we have had intensive research, documentation, and theorizing about HIV and AIDS prevention, about impact, care, stigma, discrimination, treatment, and adherence. Massive information has been produced and is still being produced. Nothing has been more attested to than the link between HIV and AIDS and injustice.

The majority of those among us who are affected belong to the most powerless members of our world who are denied power to have access to property, access to stable economies, power to make decisions and implement them, and power to control their own bodies. Thus, HIV and AIDS has for us become an apocalyptic text that vividly displays the structures of injustice and suffering, and more urgently underlines the need for justice to be served to all members of the earth community. We have been rudely reminded that a world of inequality is basically an unhealthy world.

It goes without saying that an HIV+ church is, and must be, a prophetic church that calls for justice to be served to the poor and marginalized, women, children, orphans, homosexuals, drug addicts, and sex workers. A prophetic theology in the HIV and AIDS context must expose the national and international structures of injustice and call for justice to be served to and with all.

An HIV+ church seeks a positive world by proclaiming the sacredness of all creation—that all life is sacred, hence worthy of preservation. An HIV+ church seeks a positive world, a world that affirms all human beings as created in God's image, hence worthy of dignity and presentation.[17] An HIV and AIDS positive world seeks in a practical way to put its hands on building and serving justice to all its members.

By becoming a prophetic church, we acknowledge that compassion is active. It must move the church (Mark 1:42–43; Matt 20:29–34). The transformative energy of compassion does not call upon an HIV+ positive church to merely sit, watch, and cry in pain for the suffering and the pain of one another. A compassionate church is active. Hence, being com-

---

17. Bongmba, *Facing a Pandemic*, 95–130.

passionate communities must always *move us to actively seek change*, to identify the root causes of pain, to end the pain, the suffering, the oppression, the exploitation, and the hurting with those who are most affected.

The church as a compassionate community is, therefore, not a *charitable community*, it is a *revolutionary community that seeks lasting change*. That compassion is revolutionary means that compassion is justice-seeking—it aims at tackling the root causes of suffering instead of merely addressing the symptoms of suffering. In the words of Sally B. Purvis, compassion should be "an important source of the energy we need to respond—to right the wrongs."[18] Compassionate communities, in other words, should always be involved in activism and in liberation from all forms of oppression. Such a role cannot be over-emphasized for the injustice-driven HIV and AIDS crisis.

Moreover, an HIV+ church, as a lamenting and prophetic church, must begin by serving justice within its boundaries, among its members, communities and countries. An HIV+ church, as a compassionate community, can no longer entertain patriarchy, which is a major driving force behind the spread of HIV.[19] A compassionate church must be the first to serve justice by taking concrete action to dismantle patriarchy and to empower women and all other disempowered members of the society. Within its own boundaries, an HIV+ church has no space for HIV stigma and discrimination; it has no space for the exploitation and dispossession of orphaned children and widows; it has no space for denial of affordable ARV—for the earth and everything in it belongs to the Lord.

A compassionate church also works with other justice seeking organizations for justice to be served. Let this be known: Churches that harbor those forces of oppression that propel HIV and AIDS, such as gender inequality and stigma, are not compassionate communities, hence are not effective in dismantling HIV. They are more willing to sugarcoat, to address "symptoms," rather than root causes—they are part of the problem.

TASK FOR ACADEMIC THEOLOGIANS AND RESEARCHERS

There is always more that could be said. But it suffices to say that there is quite a task ahead for professional theologians in their journeys with the church that continues to seek the realization of its call to be a

---

18. Purvis, "Compassion," 52.
19. *Report on the Global*, 21.

compassionate community—a community that embraces its HIV status as positive.[20] By positive in this context, I mean that we are a church that fully acknowledges that we are living with HIV and AIDS and we are not caught up in silence, indifference, stigmatization and discrimination. Rather we are caught up in the transformative space of compassion, which is an active state of hope and resurrection.

Our academic theologians around the world have been doing a lot to create the space where compassionate communities can be realized.[21] Yet there is still quite a lot of work to be done in this journey of becoming. We need more work on interrogating masculinities and HIV and AIDS and on theories of constructing life-affirming masculinities. The voices of children and people with disability need to be at the fore of constructing compassionate communities.

Moreover, we need our academic and church theologians, together with their students, to document for us just how much the church has managed to become a listening church that has allowed itself to be fully transformed into a compassionate community that embraces its status of being an HIV+ church. Theological researchers and educators need to assist us in analyzing the curriculum of the church and its transformation within the past twenty-six years:

Do sermons and Sunday school contents indicate an increasingly constructive engagement with HIV and AIDS? Do churches increasingly and constructively talk about sexuality? Are churches occupying the prophetic space? Are the lamentations of the church heard? What are the emerging theologies of hope and life? Does a condom have a place in the church now? Is the church a space of healing and, if so, how? What are the emerging theologies of life? What are the practical projects that are undertaken by the church to birth and nurture justice?

Premarital abstinence from sex is a major strategy of prevention in the church. How effective is that strategy and how can it be further improved? Church leaders are expected to deal competently with HIV and AIDS. Do they have sufficient training, who trains them, and how can they be further empowered? Does the laity have sufficient materials

---

20. Dube, "Theological Challenges," 523–49; Dube, *HIV/AIDS*; Maluleke, "Towards an HIV/AIDS," 59–76; "Theological Education," 105–30; Ackermann, "HIV- and AIDS," 46–50.

21. Bongmba, *Facing a Pandemic*; Phiri et al., *African women*; Phiri and Nadar, "Introduction"; Chitando, *Living with Hope*.

for Sunday school? What needs to be improved? What training is needed by the clergy and the laity? Academic theologians and researchers have a great task to evaluate just how much the church has progressed; to highlight the gaps in documentation of the voices of those among us who are affected and infected, in providing the training and in producing relevant materials in these and many other areas.

Yet academic theologians, researchers and their students also need to assess themselves in this journey of birthing compassionate communities. We need to ask ourselves: How many courses, full-time and part-time, have we created to facilitate further conversations and training of/with the church clergy and the laity? Do we now have programs such as certificate, diploma, master's, or doctorate in HIV and AIDS theological studies? How many books, conferences and workshops have we been organizing as academic theologians and researchers on HIV and AIDS in the past twenty-six years? How many research activities have been sponsored by academic departments? How about the large-scale projects that we sometimes undertake? What are the effective means that we have adopted to ensure that dissemination of our findings reach and empower our worshiping communities?

Sometimes the gap between academic theologians and researchers is a major hindrance. And what about the next twenty-six years of living and doing theology in an HIV-positive world? What are our visions and plans? We need to be more concrete and persistent in this journey of birthing compassionate communities. For, we have been informed that we need long terms plans on living with HIV and AIDS for the next quarter of a century. I believe these are some of the issues that should be on the agenda of academic theologians and researchers of the church.

AN HIV POSITIVE CHRISTOLOGY AND RADICAL SELF-IDENTIFICATION

I have, so far, drawn greatly from the body metaphor (1 Cor 12:26b) as fundamental to birthing nurturing and compassionate faith communities. I dwelled on the body metaphor, for it is a community metaphor and we live in the earth community as people (1 John 4:20–21). Yet the body metaphor is Christological as well. As I said earlier on, proclaiming that the church is HIV+ is Christological grounded theology, as well—a frame of reference that I will briefly expound.

On Being an HIV-positive Church

As the body of Christ, the church must, like its founder, identify with those who are suffering (Matt 25:31–46). Indeed, during his lifetime Jesus was mostly found with the poor and marginalized members of his society, to the extent that his fellow teachers even complained (Matt 9:10–13). He also taught and called for neighborly and caring communities (Luke 10:25–37). But perhaps the passage that most forcefully enjoins the church to occupy its identity as an HIV-positive church is Matthew 25:31–46. The narrative context of the passage is judgment. Jesus was talking about the criteria that will be employed to evaluate if one lived a worthy Christian life in order to qualify to enter the kingdom of heaven. And what is the criterion that he put forward? It is living as compassionate communities towards all the suffering and the needy in our earth communities.

What is most impressive is the manner in which Christ enjoined his followers to be compassionate. He states that he would say to those being judged in the last day: "I was hungry (…) I was thirsty (…) I was a stranger (…) naked (…) sick and in prison and you did not visit me" (Matt 25:42–43). What happens in and through this articulation is that Christ does not separate himself from the marginalized, the oppressed and the vulnerable of this world. Rather, he embodies and personifies all the suffering, marginalized, powerless, and oppressed people of the world.

I would like to name this stance as the radical self-identification of Christ. This radical self-identification must be noted since he intends to underline in no uncertain terms that Christians cannot be a church of Christ if they are not compassionate communities that radically identify with all who are suffering, marginalized and powerless in the world. In the HIV-positive world, we cannot be a church of Jesus Christ if we do not proclaim and in practice claim our Christian identity of being an HIV-positive church—a compassionate community that fully participates in suffering and earnestly seeks to foster the resurrection of everyone.

Christ's radical self-identification is gender-inclusive. It is notable that Jesus, a male, chose this self-identification. Indeed, in the story of the Good Samaritan (Luke 10:25–37), Jesus chooses a male character to demonstrate good neighborliness as being moved by compassion. I believe this is an instructive deconstruction of the gender-oppressive ethics of care that are found in many societies.

In particular, women, girls and grandmother have come to carry an unacceptable and impoverishing burden of care in the HIV and AIDS context. Compassionate communities consist of men and women who are moved into radical self-identification, including giving care to the sick. I remember Congo Brazzaville, back in 2003. I had gone to run a workshop on a theology of compassion for the churches of Central Africa. Sixty-six church leaders had been gathered from the Central African Republic, the Democratic Republic of Congo, Gabon, Cameroon, Rwanda and Congo Brazzaville.

Shortly after I gave a central-concept paper on compassion, we broke for tea. Just as I was picking my cup for tea, one church leader said something to me in French. I asked, "What did he say?" My translator explained, he says, "Compassion is for women!" I was quite annoyed and dissed back, saying,:

> Yes you are right. And, you know, the church is female. As a member of the church you are a woman. So go ahead, and be compassionate.

In Christ's radical self-identification, let us note one more aspect—namely, that the gates of granting compassion are wide open—beyond the confines of one's immediate faith community and country. That is, when we ask: "Where and to whom should we offer compassion?" the answer is: Whenever we encounter any person who is marginalized and suffering—the sick, the thirsty, the hungry, the homeless, the imprisoned, the injured, etc. (Luke 10:25–37). When we encounter any such marginalized and suffering person we must be moved by compassion and identify with them, for to ignore them is to ignore Christ. This boundless radical self-identification leaves no room for compassion denied. Compassion denied is unacceptable godlessness (Luke 18:1–8). To deny it is a failure to be church and a failure to serve Christ.

The wide open gates of compassion take us back to creation. In the story of creation we are challenged to realize that the whole of creation is sacred, that all people are fundamentally made in God's image (Gen 1:27–28) regardless of the race, gender, class, age, ethnicity, religion, disability, sexuality, and health status. Therefore, nothing will ever make any individual undeserving of compassion; for, their human dignity is guaranteed by the fact that they are created in God's image.[22]

---

22. Bongmba, *Facing a Pandemic*, 95–130.

Indeed when God's own child was sent to take the human form, this was itself a powerful articulation of compassion[23] and the radical self-identification of a God becoming a human being and dwelling among us (John 1:1–18; 3:16). This is the core of the Christian identity and practice. Compassion is therefore not an option. We are an HIV+ church. We are a compassionate community—and one that must never seek to fully live out the implication of the identity of radical-self identification with "the Other," who must never be othered.

---

23. Isaak, "The Compassionate God," 135–37.

2

The Body of Christ Has HIV

Susanne Rappmann

AT AN ECUMENICAL SERVICE in 1989, Ron Russel-Coons preached on the theme of "We have AIDS."[1] His purpose was, among other things, to call the audience's attention to the fact that HIV does not stop at the church door. We must understand that AIDS is present in all types of congregations, said Russel-Coons. It is not an illness that only afflicts "the Other," but concerns us all. We need to understand that the body of Christ has AIDS. *We* have AIDS.

I don't know if Russel-Coons was the first to use the expression, "the body of Christ has AIDS." But his sermon was widely disseminated because he was at that time part of an ecumenical committee in the United States that was reflecting on the Christian churches' position on HIV and AIDS and related issues.

One concrete result of the committee's work was a book entitled, *The Church with Aids: Renewal in the midst of crisis,* which included Russel-Coons's 1989 sermon. Several of the other contributors to the book refer to his conception of the church as the body of Christ with AIDS; and since the start of the 1990s, that and similar expressions have appeared more frequently in church documents and theological texts dealing with HIV and AIDS.[2]

But what does it really mean, "the body of Christ has AIDS?" or "the body of Christ has HIV?" Does the expression possess theological substance, or is it merely an evocative slogan? I have analyzed a number of texts and documents in which the authors have used the expression

---

1. Russell-Coons, "We have AIDS," 35–44.

2. Cf. Lutheran World Federation's statement, "Compassion." The expression is also used by other church groups, including the Catholic Church in South Africa. See Simmermacher, "Body of Christ."

in connection with descriptions or discussions of what the church is or ought to be. It is a limited body of material, but it nevertheless indicates that "the body of Christ has HIV" is a useful expression for anyone who wishes to reflect self-critically on the role of the church during a time when a pandemic of HIV and AIDS is raging.

This paper discusses some of the insights that theologians have gained through use of the expression, "the body of Christ has HIV." Those insights are summarized with the help of two key words: *solidarity* and *resurrection*. The discussion is based on Avery Dulles's ideas about the utility of models for the work of theology.[3] Such a model can provide a useful framework for better understanding both the contents and function of the expression.

Before focusing on the question of which meanings may be conveyed by "the body of Christ has HIV," I will devote a few words to the formulation of the expression. This will also provide an opportunity to say something about Dulles's theory.

THEOLOGICAL MODELS

The expression is based on a well-established image of, or metaphor for, the Christian church as the body of Christ. That image is taken from the New Testament, the epistles of St. Paul in particular, and has been widely used throughout the church's history. As have many others, St. Paul found that the human body was a useful metaphor when referring to diverse gatherings of people, in this case the church.

The human body is also used as a metaphor in other contexts—as an image of society, for example. But St. Paul does something more than employ a useful image—he adds that the church is the body of *Christ*. That additional thought enables him to develop his ecclesiology in a way that would not have been possible if he had merely referred to the church as a human body.

Thus, when theologians today broaden the metaphor of Christ's body to include affliction with HIV and AIDS, it is not the first time in history that the meaning of a well-established image has been stretched. If there is any difference, it may lie in the fact that there is now greater awareness of the utility of metaphors and models in the work of theology than there was during earlier periods of church history.

---

3. Dulles, *Models of the Church*.

Among those who have contributed to an increased understanding of that usefulness is Avery Dulles, whose now-classic work, *Models of the Church*, is of particular interest in this context. In that book, Dulles precisely describes several alternative models of the church. Based on those descriptions he clarifies the differences and similarities between, and the strengths and weaknesses of, the ecclesiologies that the models represent. An important element of Dulles's theory is that no single model can explain the phenomenon of the church. Different models emphasize different aspects, and the relevance of each varies with time and cultural context.

Inspired by Dulles, I have chosen to regard the expression, "the body of Christ has HIV" as an ecclesiological model. Among models of that category, Dulles distinguishes two basic types: explanatory and exploratory.[4]

An *explanatory model* is used to bring together everything that is known about the phenomenon to be described. An ecclesiological example might be "the church as the people of God." The advantages of this model are that it is capable of gaining acceptance due to its biblical origins, it is well-represented in the Christian tradition, and is still today regarded as useful for many Christians when speaking of their faith.

An *exploratory model*, according to Dulles, is more experimental and can lead to new theological insights. As an example he takes the model, "the church as servant." This model also has biblical origins, but its use is fairly recent in church history. In our time, however, it has proven useful for discovering aspects of the church and the Gospel that went unnoticed by earlier generations of Christians.[5]

Dulles's distinction raises the question of how to regard "the body of Christ has AIDS." Is it an explanatory or an exploratory model? The answer to that question, as we shall see, is not self-evident. It is my view that the distinction is more valuable in this context if it is used to highlight various aspects or functions of the model, than if it is perceived as a requirement to categorize the model as either explanatory or exploratory. By itself, "the body of Christ" is very much an explanatory model of the church. But the addition of HIV and AIDS shifts its function in a more experimental direction, where new theological ideas can emerge.

---

4. Dulles, *Models of the Church*, 24–25.
5. Dulles, *Models of the Church*, 26.

SOLIDARITY

For the writers who began to use the concept of "the body of Christ has HIV" during the late 1980s and early 1990s, the purpose was to arouse awareness within the church. It was also to demonstrate solidarity with victims of HIV and AIDS and provide a response to the sort of theology which proclaims that HIV and AIDS is a divine punishment. All that became possible through theological reflections on the ecclesiological model, "the body of Christ has HIV."

Based on that model, it was possible to argue that all members of the church are part of a larger whole. The membership that comes with baptism also confers fellowship with Christ, the body's head, and with all the other parts of the body. On the basis of St. Paul's conception of the body and the interdependence of its parts, it could be argued that, if some members of the church have HIV and AIDS, it is a fact that concerns us all. St. Paul also provided support for belief in the importance of solidarity with parts of the body that appear to be weak, and of members to share in each other's suffering.

The essence of the model was, to begin with, relatively conventional; and based on Dulles's theory. I understand it to be mainly explanatory. But with the passage of time, as the spread of HIV and AIDS accelerates and writers increasingly adopt "the body of Christ has HIV," the model will give rise to new ideas. These, however, are likely to be clearly related to established interpretations of the church as the body of Christ.

Among recent interpretations are those which deal with the church's relationship to human sexuality. That is a burning issue in this context, due to the fact that one of the HI virus's most common channels of infection is via sexual relations. Referring to the model of the church as a body, several writers have drawn attention to the fact that the church's membership consists of sexual beings. Accordingly, sexuality cannot be regarded as solely a private matter, but something that concerns our common existence. Today, when 40 million people are contaminated with HIV, the church has to realize that it is time to break the silence! By avoiding an open discussion of sexuality, the church is contributing to the spread of the pandemic, and also to the stigmatization and social exclusion of HIV and AIDS victims.[6] These consequences are hardly compatible with the model of the church expressed by "the body of Christ has HIV."

---

6. Ackermann, "Tamar's Cry," 45.

When the standpoint of the church is formulated, it is essential to seriously reflect upon what it means to be a moral community. According to Denise Ackermann, the sexual morality that is most often preached by the church is oversimplified and ignores the complex nature of human existence. Research has clearly shown that the HIV and AIDS pandemic is intimately connected with problems of poverty and gender inequality. If the church does not include these issues in its reflections on what it means for humans to live together—and instead insists that the principal means of preventing the spread of HIV is to abstain from sex before marriage and to remain sexually faithful to one's spouse thereafter—it is almost certain to do more harm than good.

For Ackermann, the model of the church as "the HIV-infected body of Christ" provides a useful framework within which to reflect on sexuality, and also to discuss what it means to be part of a community whose members are dependent on each other. She maintains that it is essential for the community's ethics to be founded on principles of justice and equality. With such a moral platform, the church would be well equipped to encounter all those within and outside the church who are afflicted with HIV and AIDS.

At first glance, "the body of Christ has HIV" may seem like a rather limited model for addressing the church's relationship to HIV and AIDS issues. It entails a risk that theological reflections will be concerned primarily with internal matters. But the texts that I have analyzed also contain important incentives to deal with matters outside the church.

A common line of thought is that, if the church is Christ's body in the world today, it must act as Jesus did. He often moved among people on the margins of society, including the sick and the reviled. The image of the church as an HIV-infected body may therefore be regarded as a body/community in solidarity with all those who suffer in various ways—from sickness, stigmatization, poverty, or oppression.[7]

RESURRECTION

HIV and AIDS is inevitably associated with suffering and death, and it is therefore not surprising that theologians use "the body of Christ has HIV" when addressing issues of solidarity and suffering. More remarkable, perhaps, is that the model has led to a renewal of reflections on the

---

7. Cf. Dube "Theological Challeges."

resurrection of Christ (although the resurrection is a theme that also appears in texts of St. Paul which evoke the image of Christ's body).

Letty Russel is among those who have pointed out the need to reflect on church teachings regarding the body's resurrection and eternal life. It is crucial, however, that such reflection lead not to a flight from the reality of life's tragedies, but to the formulation of a theology in which the resurrection expresses God's "No!" to evil, suffering, and death.[8]

Within that perspective, what hope is there for an HIV-infected body? What hope can the HIV-infected church offer? The realization that the church is itself afflicted is an important starting point for the majority of the texts I have analyzed. When we understand that the church is an infected body, we can also begin to conceive what it means that Christ identified that body with his own. Our hope is based on the fact that Christ himself conveyed his body through death to resurrected life. Death and misfortune have never been the last words of the Christian faith;[9] but that does not mean denial of life's trials and troubles.

Musa W. Dube takes the model of the church as an HIV-infected body as her point of departure for a discussion of how the church can serve as a countervailing force at a time when the HIV and AIDS pandemic is one of the factors that threaten the functioning of human communities.[10] For Dube, the church as the body of Christ is a vibrant community with a message of life—and, indeed, of life in abundance. This does not change if the body has HIV; rather, that condition is an occasion for solidarity with the afflicted. The crucified Christ is present in our midst. This is an important observation; but even more important is the church's task of proclaiming the resurrection of Christ. And that resurrection, according to Dube, is an expression of God's "No!" to all social injustices that lead to the suffering and death of humans.

It is clear that, for Dube, the model of "the body of Christ has HIV" functions to a great extent in an explanatory manner. Based on the established interpretation of the church as a community of solidarity, she is able to critically analyze unjust structures, both within and outside the church, that lead to death. The consequences which she elucidates do not

---

8. Russel, "Re-Imagining the Bible," 201–10.
9. Ackermann, "Tamar's Cry," 51–52.
10. Dube, "Theological Challenges," 535–49.

conform with the image of the church as the body of the crucified and resurrected.

But the fact that a writer uses a model to explore new theological ground does not prevent its also being used in an explanatory fashion. That is what several writers do, I have found, when they focus on the significance of Holy Communion for the church's members. In their writings, there is a clear attempt to maintain the unity of suffering and hope, life and death, crucifixion, and resurrection.

One example is provided by Denise Ackermann, who points out that Holy Communion was instituted on the night that Jesus was betrayed, and is thereby deeply rooted in the problems and tragedies of human life. Holy Communion involves a sharing of exposure to misfortune. It is a rite that is based on solidarity, the breaking and sharing of bread, in which all members are regarded as co-equals. But according to Ackermann, Holy Communion is also a communal meal that crosses boundaries; for, among the participants are those who have died. It is a meal of hope that heralds the perfection of creation—a time or situation in which the church is no longer a body infected with HIV or sick with AIDS, but has become what it and its members are ordained to be.

THE BODY OF CHRIST HAS HIV

It has been very interesting to analyze texts that include the expression, "the body of Christ has AIDS" and "the body of Christ has HIV." But I must acknowledge that it has also been difficult, because there is something like a chasm between the reality described by many of the writers and the reality that I encounter as theologian and priest.

Based on her experience of South Africa, for example, Denise Ackermann writes:

> Attending funerals every weekend is a numbing task. It is more than numbing when the church as the Body of Christ itself feels amputated as its members fill coffins.[11]

It seems appropriate to conclude that the value of "the body of Christ has HIV" as an ecclesiological model depends on where in the world one happens to be located. It is a conclusion that also follows from Dulles's theory regarding the utility of models for the work of theology. Likewise,

---

11. Ackermann, "Tamar's Cry," 30–31.

it is interesting to note that the expression has been perceived as relevant in a wide variety of contexts—from U.S. gay churches in the 1980s, to the community of Lutheran bishops in Southern Africa in the current decade.

How, then, does all this affect my role as minister to a Lutheran congregation in Mölndal, a medium-size Swedish town? Is "the body of Christ has HIV" a useful model for the church and its manner of relating to the global HIV epidemic? Let me begin my response by noting something that is obvious, but perhaps just for that reason needs to be mentioned: The model cannot by itself explain or be used to explore the essence of the church, and I cannot see that any of the theological writings that I have analyzed applies the model in either way.

But I find that it has great value as one image among others. It is a robust model because, among other things, it is rooted in the established ecclesiological model of the church as the body of Christ. That model contains the seeds of various interpretations that provide a basis for many lines of further development, including everything from conceptions of the body and sexuality to Holy Communion and eschatology.

For the majority of my congregation, HIV and AIDS is not something that is part of everyday life. Thus, there is a risk that those who are afflicted may feel themselves rejected. In order to make the existence of HIV and AIDS visible, even in my town, I see a value in using the expression, "the body of Christ has HIV." It certainly arouses attention!

But the value of this ecclesiological model is much greater. It reminds me that my congregation and I are part of something much larger—a global fellowship. I am part of a fellowship that extends over space and time, with the parts and the whole dependent on each other. When someone suffers, I am also affected.

Based on the insights that theologians have reached through use of the model, I have become painfully aware that I am among those who are not actively helping to prevent the further spread of the disease. The injustices of the world, including poverty and gender inequality, are phenomena that we humans have created and maintain—and which are therefore in our power to change.

The self-critical question I pose is: What can the church and I as an individual do within our local spheres to actively help to prevent the further spread of HIV? It is, of course, a question to which there are many answers that would require a lifetime to complete. But by its very utterance, the question demonstrates that "the body of Christ has HIV" is an expression that is as relevant in Sweden as anywhere else. It gives rise to self-critical reflection on the manner in which the church and I myself relate to churches around the world.

In addition, I find that the reflections on the body and sexuality which have arisen from the model are useful in my daily life; for even here in quiet Mölndal, violence against women is a frequent occurrence, and is just as frequently buried with silence. Likewise I have found that theological reflections on the resurrection are valuable in my encounters with the gravely ill and the dying. The hope that emerges from those reflections is simple, but does not ignore the darker realities of life and death.

It is also a hope that demands action! The body of Christ has HIV. What are we going to do about that?

3

Jesus, the Leper, and HIV and AIDS: Suffering, Solidarity, and Structural Transformation

Kenneth R. Overberg, S.J.

HIV AND AIDS RAISE ethical questions that extend throughout the life cycle and around the globe. The Hebrew and Christian scriptures and the social teaching/human rights tradition provide the foundations of a response to these questions. A brief story highlights the systemic issues, rooted in structures of sin that facilitate the spread of HIV. Lament, action, and trust make up the appropriate elements of a concrete response to the question "What ought I/we to do?" and point to the profound age-old challenge, the mystery of God and suffering.

BIBLICAL AND ETHICAL FOUNDATIONS

Deeply embedded in some streams of Hebrew thought is the sense that good deeds lead to blessing and evil deeds to suffering. If a person were experiencing sickness or other trials, then that person must have sinned in the past. This perspective is grounded in the Deuteronomy tradition, and is perfectly expressed by Job's "friends" (see the series of speeches in chapters 3–31). The Book of Job, however, challenges this tradition; Job suffers despite his innocence (Job 31 especially).[1]

Jesus too challenges this belief. In the exquisite scene described in chapter nine of John's Gospel, Jesus heals a blind man. Then threats, excuses, and faith take center stage. Even before the healing, Jesus declares that the man's blindness was not due to his or his parents' sin (John 9:2–5). Neither Job nor Jesus explains away the pain of suffering, but neither views sickness or other trials as a punishment from God.[2]

---

1. Harrington, *Why Do We Suffer?* 15–49; see also Gutierrez, *On Job*.
2. Moloney, *Gospel of John*, 289–99; Brown, *Gospel According to John*, 369–82; see also Dewey, *Word in Time*, 16–18.

Leprosy was one of those diseases that many interpreted as God's punishment. The Book of Leviticus devotes two chapters (13 and 14) to discussing this condition. The harsh rules describe an image familiar to the imaginations of many of us:

> The person who has the leprous disease shall wear torn clothes and let the hair of his head be dishevelled; and he shall cover his upper lip and cry out, "Unclean, unclean." He shall remain unclean as long as he has the disease; he is unclean. He shall live alone; his dwelling shall be outside the camp. (13:45–46)

Certainly, ancient peoples were afraid of contagion, but for the people of Israel leprosy became a ritual impurity more than a medical problem.[3] They considered it divine punishment and feared that the community would also suffer if the leper were not forced "outside the camp."

Jesus not only rejects the judgment (John 9:3) but also crosses the boundaries of purity laws to touch the alienated. Mark's Gospel describes the scene this way:

> A leper came to him begging him, and kneeling he said to him, "If you choose, you can make me clean." Moved with pity, Jesus stretched out his hand and touched him, and said to him, "I do choose. Be made clean!" Immediately the leprosy left him, and he was made clean. (1:40–42)

With a simple but profound touch, Jesus breaks down barriers, challenges customs and laws that alienate, embodies his convictions about the inclusive meaning of the reign of God.

This event reveals not only Jesus' care for an individual in need but also his concern about structures of society. Jesus steps across the boundaries separating the unclean and actually touches the leper. In doing so, Jesus enters into the leper's isolation and becomes unclean. Human care and compassion direct Jesus' action. He calls into question the purity code that alienates and oppresses people already in need. Indeed, this encounter with the leper is one example of how Jesus reaches out to the marginal people in Jewish society, whether they are women, the possessed, or lepers.

The scene also reveals Jesus' recognition of the Biblical conviction that faith must be connected with politics, economics, and all structures

---

3. Faley, "Leviticus," 69–70; Mull and Sandquist Mull, "Biblical Leprosy," 32–39 and 62; see also Crossan, *Jesus*, 77–84.

Jesus, the Leper, and HIV and AIDS

of society. His encounter with the leper is one example, but Jesus also embodied and expressed this vision in his parables about God's reign and in his healings and table fellowship.[4]

Today many people living with HIV and AIDS experience judgment, stigmatization, and rejection—just like the leper. In ways subtle and not so subtle, they too are forced "outside the camp," whether it be housing, employment, insurance, school, or even religion. Other societal powers make the situation worse. Throughout the world, economic systems and decisions trap people in poverty. Racism fosters oppression. Religions promote judgmental attitudes. Violence and widespread denial of any real freedom force women into tragic situations. All these situations provide the perfect conditions for the spread of HIV.

How are we to respond? Clearly, our Scriptures challenge us to live as faithful disciples of Jesus. Our biblical reflections have led us to three specific points that guide responses to HIV and AIDS. 1) We resist the temptation to judge and condemn people. HIV and AIDS are not punishment sent by God. This change of attitude is where we start. 2) We respond with care and compassion to those infected and affected by HIV, crossing the boundaries of fear and prejudice. With the attitude of Jesus, we reach out to these sisters and brothers. 3) We recognize the need for societal change as well as individual behavioral change. This too means action—systemic action. Such a response accepts personal responsibility to challenge and change political platforms, economic strategies, and governmental decisions that foster a culture of oppression and death.

Key themes from liberation theology and the social teachings of our churches offer a moral vision that offers direction for action concerning the AIDS crisis.[5] These themes are human dignity, solidarity, justice, and the common good. (In the Catholic Church in the United States, these key ideas have been linked together in a comprehensive ethical system, the consistent ethic of life, first articulated by Cardinal Joseph Bernardin more than twenty years ago.)[6]

Human dignity is the foundation of all the social teachings.[7] Because all human beings are created in God's image, we are sacred and precious.

---

4. Dewey, *Word in Time*, 110–12 and passim; Schillebeeckx, *Jesus*, 179–271; Meier, "Jesus," 1318–28.

5. Sobrino, *Where Is God?*; Himes, *Modern Catholic*; "Towards a Policy."

6. Bernardin, *Consistent Ethic*; Bernardin, *A Moral Vision*.

7. John XXIII, "Peace on Earth," 201–41; Vatican II, "Church in the Modern," 243–335; "Nurturing Peace."

Accordingly, all persons have worth and dignity, rooted simply in who they are (and not in what they do or achieve). Situations that limit or undermine human dignity cry out for change. All forms of discrimination are wrong, whether in housing, jobs, insurance, health care, or religion.

Technology and globalization constantly remind us of the deeper interdependence—our shared humanity—of the human family. Many of Pope John Paul II's writings emphasized this solidarity, especially with the poor of the world.[8] He affirmed that Christians follow God in expressing a preferential option for the poor. This option recognizes the power of economic and social structures to perpetuate poverty and limit personal freedom, harming both those who oppress and those who are oppressed.

Justice, right relationships along with the structural recognition of human dignity and rights and responsibilities, is another major theme emphasized throughout the social teachings. Action on behalf of justice and participation in the transformation of the world has been called "a constitutive dimension of the preaching of the gospel."[9]

The goal of justice is to create a global society where the common good flourishes. The common good means all those things necessary for all peoples to live truly human lives.[10] What most of us take for granted—food, water, clothing, shelter, sanitation, appropriate health care, participation in politics—is lacking in the lives of hundreds of millions of the human family.

The moral vision grounded in Scripture and these four themes recognizes that politics, media, money, and class—and not our faith—may well be the real source of our values. So it offers a profoundly challenging framework for responding to the ethical dilemmas of HIV and AIDS.

GLOBAL STRUCTURAL ISSUES

HIV and AIDS raise ethical questions that extend throughout the life cycle and around the globe. These questions cluster in five areas. The first is focused on birth, infancy, and childhood; issues include preventing HIV transmission from mother to child, abortion, and caring for AIDS

---

8. John Paul II, *On Social Concern*; Kammer, *Doing Faithjustice*, 121–60, 181–87; Sniegocki, "Social Ethics," 7–32; "On the Situation."

9. Synod of Bishops, "Justice in the World," 514 (#6); "Statement on Latin America."

10. John XXIII, "Peace on Earth," 213–16 (#53–66); "What Does God Require"; see also Kobia, "Epiphany 2007 Message."

Jesus, the Leper, and HIV and AIDS

orphans. The second cluster relates to HIV-infected persons and their relationships; issues include informing partners, decisions by discordant couples (when one person is HIV-positive and the other is not), and dealing with health-care providers. A third cluster looks at end-of-life issues and a fourth the responsibilities of society including HIV-testing, education, and prevention programs. The fifth cluster, the focus of this section, centers on the economic and social and political structures that contribute to behaviors that facilitate the spread of HIV. Poverty, racism, oppression of women, globalization and the maximization of profits, forced migration, war, and violence of all kinds create the perfect breeding grounds for the growth of the HIV and AIDS epidemic. Most if not all of the questions in the first four clusters are influenced and even created by these global structural issues. To confront the AIDS pandemic adequately, then, demands addressing these often overwhelming problems that can rightly be called "structures of sin."[11]

A Story

Clearly, we do not have space here to address all these issues. One woman's story, however, embodies many of these forces. And this one story symbolizes millions.[12] Nsanga, a woman in her twenties with two children, had been married to a schoolteacher. Because of structural adjustment measures instituted by the International Monetary Fund (IMF), the government of Zaire (now the Democratic Republic of Congo) was forced to make cutbacks in its expenses, including laying off teachers and health workers. Nsanga's husband lost his job, was not able to find a new one, began spending their small resources on drinking, and finally simply disappeared. Nsanga was very poor, as were her living conditions.

> [She lived in a] single room which was part of a corrugated-roofed block surrounding an open courtyard. The yard contained a shared water tap, a roofless bathing stall, and a latrine, but no electricity. In good weather Nsanga and her neighbors moved their charcoal stoves outdoors to cook. In the courtyard, they also washed dishes and clothes and prepared vegetables for the pot. Wastewater ran out to an open ditch outside. Like the yard, the street was unpaved, deeply rutted, muddy in the rainy season, and dusty in the dry months. Mosquitoes were ubiquitous in the neighborhood, and

---

11. John Paul II, *Gospel of Life*, 26 (#12); "Called to be the One Church."
12. Nsanga's story is taken from Schoepf, "Health, Gender Relations," 153–68.

malaria and diarrheal diseases were common causes of death in young children. Many families ate only one meal per day and children were especially undernourished. Many people had deep, hacking coughs that suggested pulmonary tuberculosis.[13]

Nsanga, like most poor women in Kinshasa (the capital city with a population of several million people), had only a few years of education in primary school. She unsuccessfully tried to find employment and so did small jobs in the neighborhood. These were not enough to pay for rent and food, so Nsanga began exchanging sex for subsistence. For a year, her lover was a married man who paid her rent. After she became pregnant, he left her, so Nsanga had to find more partners. At the time, the "neighborhood rate was equivalent to U.S. fifty cents per brief encounter,"[14] so two partners per day would produce about $30 a month.

Nsanga's medical history included an earlier ectopic pregnancy that led to a blood transfusion. She had symptoms of a sexually transmitted disease but had no money to consult a doctor. Condoms were for "prostitutes" and she was not one of those but only a mother trying to fulfill her obligations.

> Abandonment, divorce, and widowhood force many women who are without other resources into commercial sex work. In the presence of HIV, however, this survival strategy has been transformed into a death strategy.[15]

Nsanga's story points to the pervasive power of poverty. It also highlights the impact of socioeconomic and political conditions, including the consequences of IMF policies and the cultural oppression of women. Already facing poverty, Nsanga and her family turn from a difficult life to face a tragic one when her husband loses his job as a school teacher. Marriage and family begin to unravel, the result of the country's national debt and the IMF's structural adjustment policies. The cutbacks in education and health care that came from budget pressures lead finally to death and the destruction of this family. Political and economic structures combine with already existing poverty, oppression of women, and lack of education to facilitate the growth of the AIDS pandemic.

---

13. Schoepf, "Health, Gender Relations," 157–58.
14. Schoepf, "Health, Gender Relations," 159.
15. Schoepf, "Health, Gender Relations," 160.

Jesus, the Leper, and HIV and AIDS

War and Other Violence

For millions of others, such a situation is made even worse by war or forced migration. Ethnic and religious conflicts, genocide, and the many forms of violence connected with wars are major contributors to the spread of HIV. Refugee camps have become perfect breeding grounds for HIV and AIDS. Rape is used as a weapon of war, not only as violence but as an attempt to destroy the bonds of family and community. Ironically, even the presence of peacekeeping forces can lead to higher rates of HIV infection.

Wars, including numerous civil wars, have created millions of refugees, many of them women and children. All forms of forced migration, whether because of wars, economics, or natural disasters, lead to a breakdown of family and community, to a loss of cultural structures and norms, to a lack of basic needs like food and shelter and education.

> HIV flourishes, particularly, in situations of hopelessness and social breakdown. HIV control demands a measure of control over one's own life, a sense of self, of self-worth, and a belief that there is a future which is worth planning for. In a refugee camp, women and children have none of these.[16]

In many countries, HIV infection rates among the military are often significantly higher than in the general population. Thus, the movement of troops, either for war or for peacekeeping or for relief work, can lead to higher infection rates, for example, among sex workers. There is the additional risk of new viral strains being introduced in all the communities.[17]

A host of other threats are part of the vicious cycles of HIV and AIDS and social structures and dynamics related to war and its impact. Some are surprisingly practical—such as the location of water supplies or latrines in the refugee camps. If these locations are too isolated, young girls and boys and women who must go to these places face an increased risk of rape. Others are profoundly human—such as seeking sex as a source of affection. Also, in "post genocide situations, sex and the desire for pregnancy may become a means for replacing lost family, community and/or ethnic group."[18]

---

16. Paterson, *Women in the Time*, 8.
17. Smith and McDonagh, *Reality of AIDS*, 113–14.
18. Smith and McDonagh, *Reality of AIDS*, 117.

Other threats are related to issues already considered, for example, poverty and the oppression of women. In conflict situations and in emergencies following natural disasters, men are usually the decision-makers and the ones controlling resources.

> Men usually control relief supplies and can barter these in exchange for women's only tradable commodity—sex.[19]

RESPONSE OF LAMENT, ACTION, TRUST

Enter our lament in your book; store every tear in your flask (see Psalm 56). The staggering suffering in our world can overwhelm us and leads spontaneously and appropriately to lament. Those who directly experience the intense suffering of HIV and AIDS surely need to lament. So must others, overcoming their numbness and acknowledging the disease and death that affect so many millions of members of the human family.

Things are not right. The first step to grief and healing is to move from overwhelmed silence to speech, the bold speech of lament. The Psalms show us how to speak out against suffering and oppression, even against God. Such crying out allows us both to grieve and to grow into a mature covenant partner with God and not merely a subservient one. Lament confronts the evils in our lives and religion and culture and world, proclaiming that these must not be.[20]

This is the fast that I wish: untying the thongs of the yoke, sharing your bread, not turning your back (see Isaiah 58:5–7). Given the complex, interwoven nature of the structural issues and given their immense impact on the spread of the AIDS pandemic, what action can we take? We can begin by recognizing the sinfulness of some of these social structures.

Recent Christian thinking has developed a

> double understanding of the dynamic of personal and structural sin: human beings structure the sinfulness into a social system or arrangement, and the system or structure coercively shapes the behavior of individuals, both those who oppress and those who are oppressed.[21]

---

19. Smith and McDonagh, *Reality of AIDS*, 117.
20. Brueggemann, "The Costly Loss," 57–71.
21. Kammer, *Doing Faithjustice*, 101–2.

Jesus, the Leper, and HIV and AIDS

Moving from theory to practice, of course, is almost always very challenging; and it is especially so in the complexity and suffering of the AIDS epidemic. Still, human dignity, solidarity, justice, and the universal common good provide profound and solid ethical foundations for life-respecting and life-saving practices.

The vicious cycles of unjust economic policies, war, poverty, and the oppression of women, as in Nsanga's story, cause dehumanization and death. The preferential option for the poor, the recognition of the feminization of poverty, the just use of scarce resources, and the growing appreciation of nonviolence offer concrete alternatives to these sinful social structures. Yet breaking into a vicious cycle is so very difficult; it seems that many actions must be taken simultaneously.[22]

Certainly, though, one key entry point is the crushing poverty experienced by so many millions of people in our world. At the structural level, a number of changes are possible. One of those changes, the relief of some international debt, has already begun. To celebrate the new millennium, many groups and individuals (including Pope John Paul II) urged the forgiveness of massive debts of some of the poorest nations. These debts, often encouraged by international institutions and incurred by corrupt leaders, continue to oppress the debtor nations, limiting and reducing health care and education. More debt forgiveness along with responsible use of their resources by local governments will further reduce poverty, promote the common good, and address AIDS directly.[23]

One practice that greatly increased debts was the purchase of weapons by governments. So arms sales promote both violence and poverty. Changing that dynamic would offer a double benefit, reducing violence and having funds to address some of the root cause of conflict and disease.[24]

Another possible economic change is the creation of free trade agreements that are fair, especially for the poor. Fair agreements will be aware of the perspective of the poor and not just the powerful.[25] The preferential

---

22. Kammer, *Doing Faithjustice*, 189–204.

23. "Debt-for-AIDS Swaps"; see also "Forgive and Forget."

24. Hartung and Berrigan, "Militarization of U.S."; see other reports at this same site; also, on this issue and others in this section, see Skylstad, "Letter to President Bush."

25. See the statement by Central American and U.S. bishops on CAFTA at http://www.wola.org/index.php?option=com_content&task=viewp&id=372&Itemid=2>; other information from a human rights perspective can also be found here (Washington Office on Latin America).

option for the poor will probably not convince many leaders of governments and corporations, but pointing out that ethical business practices are ultimately also good business practices might. Another motivation is security, as poverty nourishes not only HIV and AIDS but also terrorism. Both the possibility of seeing the world from the side of the poor and the need for different motivations and values highlight the central place for dialogue if change is to occur.

Global structures require responses from governments and international agencies. But what can individuals do? They can, of course, work in these major institutions, contributing talent and insight. Individuals can also participate in advocacy and activism that may be necessary to achieve change. Such pressure best reflects gospel values when it is nonviolent. One example of surprising success of such advocacy has been some of the licensing and pricing changes accepted by the major pharmaceutical companies (though more changes are surely necessary).[26]

Publicizing the success of nonviolent resistance and advocacy is essential. Many people instinctively slip into the age-old conviction (indeed, religion) that only violence saves. The success of nonviolence, especially in recent years, must be recognized and taught so that new attitudes may develop.[27]

What else can individuals do regarding sinful social structures? Individuals can begin by accepting responsibility to change their worldview by moving beyond many messages from their own societies to acknowledge the reality of economic and political policies and practices that oppress people. Such insight often comes from experience rather than from mere words, from contact not just concepts.[28]

Such insight leads to some kind of action. Some individuals may choose to volunteer for several years to participate with international groups attempting to meet immediate needs and to plant seeds for structural change, e.g., Peace Corps or Jesuit Volunteers International. Others may choose a career with Oxfam or Doctors Without Borders (or similar organizations). Still others may support such organizations with their donations.

26. Irwin et al., *Global AIDS*, 115–33.
27. Wink, *Engaging the Powers*, 13–31 and 243–57.
28. Kolvenbach, "The Service of Faith." For examples of Kolvenbach's point and for inspiring stories of what an individual or small group can accomplish, see *Linked for Life*.

Jesus, the Leper, and HIV and AIDS

Individuals may donate their time to advocacy groups, with the Internet offering new and creative possibilities. Surely not all aspects of the vicious cycles can be addressed by one group, but a part can be. Groups based in parishes or schools can inform others about sweatshops and promote alternative fair-trade goods. Other individuals can participate in groups addressing racism or family violence or inferior education in their cities.

Individuals can become directors of corporations and develop more just policies. At lower levels similar choices and practices can be implemented. Other individuals can work to enhance corporate responsibility through shareholder resolutions.

Individuals can vote, choosing candidates that challenge sinful structures and create alternatives. Individuals can name and critique anti-life aspects of the political parties. Individuals can run for office.

Individuals can try to live gospel values authentically in all dimensions of their lives.

Do not let your hearts be troubled; trust in God (see John 14:1). People of faith will continue to work with many others in searching in solidarity for creative and courageous ways to overcome suffering and its causes. People of faith will also bring their own particular motivation and vision, rooted in their religious beliefs. Christians are an Easter people, trusting that good overcomes evil, that life overcomes death. Ultimately, Christians will face suffering and political and economic challenges and will take action because they trust in God. This is not a pie-in-the-sky optimism, but a profound conviction about the God revealed by Jesus.

Where does such trust come from? Christians find the source of this trust in Jesus' own experience and then in the community's experience of Jesus. Scripture scholars have helped us to appreciate that at the heart of Jesus' living and dying was a loving relationship with God and a bold, creative proclamation of God's Reign.[29] Here we find the foundation of Jesus' own trust.

So Christians can help create the future by responding to the dark abyss of HIV and AIDS—to disease, death, and systemic evils—with lament, action, and profound trust in God.

---

29. Sobrino, *Christology*, 41–78; Kammer, *Doing Faithjustice*, 41–59; Hill, *Jesus, the Christ*, 42–62.

> HIV/AIDS brings with it new anguish and new terrors and anxiety, new trials of pain and endurance, new occasions for compassion. But it cannot change one enduring fact: God's love for us all.[30]

Even in the midst of AIDS' staggering suffering and systemic evils, nothing can snatch us out of God's hands.

THE MYSTERY OF GOD AND SUFFERING

Still, this profound trust often does not come easily. The pandemic's suffering continues to overwhelm individuals, communities, entire nations. Such suffering often leads people to ask about God: "Who is God?" "How can a good and gracious God allow this to happen?" "Where is God in all this suffering?" "Is there a God?" Those directly involved in suffering often ask: "Why did this happen to me?" and sometimes even "What did I do wrong to be punished in this way?"

Humans have long searched for some satisfying insights into these and similar questions. The whole Book of Job in the Bible is dedicated to this topic. Christians have focused, in particular, on the suffering and death of Jesus in the hope of discovering meaning for suffering. Some of these biblical perspectives, however, fail to satisfy contemporary hearts and minds that long for the God of compassion revealed by Jesus.

In order to penetrate more deeply into this mystery of God and suffering and to develop an understanding closer to the vision of Jesus, we first consider the life and death of Jesus, including some of the dominant interpretations of his suffering and death. We will then return to Scripture and Tradition for another perspective on Jesus' life and death, and see what this means for our image of God and how it grounds our threefold response of lament, action, and trust.

Jesus' Life and Teachings

From the Gospels, as we saw earlier, we learn three important points about Jesus and suffering: 1) Jesus resisted suffering and its personal and social causes and is frequently described healing persons; 2) Jesus rejected the conviction that suffering is the punishment for sin; 3) Jesus expressed a profound trust in a loving, compassionate, and present God.

---

30. *Called to Compassion*, 28.

Jesus, the Leper, and HIV and AIDS

First, many gospel stories tell of Jesus healing the blind and sick. Matthew's Gospel summarizes this way:

> Then Jesus went about all the cities and villages, teaching in their synagogues and proclaiming the good news of the kingdom, and curing every disease and every sickness. (9:35)

Second, in the Hebrew tradition is the conviction that suffering is punishment for sin, called the Law of Retribution.[31] The people in exile in Babylon, for example, interpreted this political-social event as God's punishment for their failure to follow the covenant faithfully. This conviction appears in many religions and cultures. Jesus, however, rejected it. Matthew's Jesus in the Sermon on the Mount describes God as showering rain on evil persons as well as good ones (Matt 5:45). Similarly, John's Jesus heals the blind man and explicitly rejects the idea that suffering is punishment for sin (John 9:1–41, especially 2–5).

Third, implicitly and explicitly the gospels reveal Jesus' intimate, loving relationship with God. Jesus' surprising use of *Abba* ("Daddy") to describe God conveys a sense of simplicity, familiarity, fidelity and trust.[32] The parables also give us a glimpse of Jesus' sense of God. The Prodigal Son (Luke 15:11–32) tells us a lot about the father, forgiving the son without any bitterness, celebrating his return, and consoling the angry older brother. *Abba* is a loving, forgiving, gentle parent. Even as he faced suffering and death, Jesus remained faithful to his call, always trusting God. In the resurrection, God confirms Jesus' faithfulness.

Interpreting a Terrible Death

The life and teaching of Jesus highlighted the healing presence of a God of love and life. In the end, however, Jesus suffered a horrible execution. The mystery of suffering and death—first Jesus' and later others'—led the early Christian communities to search for light and meaning. They looked to their culture and their Hebrew Scriptures for possible interpretations. They included these insights in their preaching and eventually in the Christian Scriptures.

From culture they knew about ransom. From their Jewish practices they also experienced sacrifice and atonement. From their Wisdom

---

31. For more details, see Harrington, *Why Do We Suffer?* 15–29.

32. Elliott, "Patronage and Clientism," 39–48; Dewey, "Truth That," 7–11; Schillebeeckx, *Jesus*, 256–71.

literature they were familiar with the theme of the vindication of the Innocent Sufferer. From the prophet Isaiah (chapters 42, 49, 50, 52–53) Jesus' followers creatively used the songs of the Suffering Servant to interpret Jesus' suffering and death. The Messiah, of course, was not expected to be a suffering messiah. The facts of crucifixion and death jarred Jesus' followers into searching the Hebrew Scriptures for insight for proclaiming and interpreting his death (see the letter to the Hebrews, for example).[33]

Scholars tell us that what the Bible understands by terms such as sacrifice and atonement may be quite different from the understandings that many of us have. For example, for Hebrew people, the blood of the sacrificed animal symbolized the life of the person or community. Pouring the blood on the altar was a symbolic gesture reuniting life with God. The sacrifices were an expression of the people's desire for reconciliation and union with God.[34]

It must be noted, however, that even while emphasizing these more positive meanings of sacrifice, most of the scholars pass over in silence the fact that the ritual still includes violence and the death of the victim—dimensions that are foreign to Jesus' vision of the reign of God.

Throughout the centuries Christians have reflected on and developed these different interpretations, leading to a variety of theologies and popular pieties, some of them quite distant from the Scriptures and even farther from the vision of Jesus.

In the fourth century, St. Augustine spoke of satisfaction for sin in legal terms of debts and justice. A key development took place in the twelfth century when the theologian St. Anselm used St. Augustine's ideas to describe atonement for sin. Anselm, reflecting the medieval culture of his day, understood sin to be something like a peasant insulting a king. Reconciliation would require satisfaction for this insult to the king's honor. Sin, however, is an infinite offense against God that demands adequate atonement. While humanity was obliged to atone, no human could pay this infinite debt. Only God could do so adequately.[35]

According to this twelfth-century view, that is exactly what Jesus, the God-Man, accomplished by his suffering and death. It was actually later theologians and preachers who added to Anselm's position by

33. Dewey, "Can We Let Jesus Die," 135–59.
34. Tambasco, *A Theology of Atonement*, 65–71.
35. Winter, *The Atonement*, 61–79; see also Cahill, "The Atonement Paradigm," 418–32.

emphasizing blood and pain as the satisfaction that placated God's anger. Most Christians still grow up with such an understanding, although some are uneasy with this view, even if they do not know why.

This image of God—angry, demanding, even bloodthirsty—often appears in sermons, songs, and popular pieties today, although the focus is usually placed on Jesus' willingness to bear the suffering. Initially, this willingness to suffer for us may seem profoundly moving and consoling. But we must ask several questions of this interpretation. What does this say about God the Father? What kind of God could demand such torture of the beloved Son? Is this the God revealed by Jesus in his words and deeds?

Jesus Is Not Plan B

There is an *alternative* interpretation of the life and death of Jesus, also expressed in the Scriptures and throughout the tradition. This view, perhaps only on the margins of many people's religious understanding and devotion, is completely orthodox. Indeed, it offers perspectives much closer to Jesus' own experience and vision.

What, briefly, is the heart of this alternative interpretation? It holds that the whole purpose of creation is for the Incarnation, God's sharing of life and love in a unique and definitive way. God becoming human is not an afterthought, an event to make up for original sin and human sinfulness. Incarnation is God's first thought, the original design for all creation. The purpose of Jesus' life is the fulfillment of the whole creative process, of God's eternal longing to become human. Theologians call this the primacy of the Incarnation.

For many of us who have lived a lifetime with the atonement view, it may be hard at first to hear this alternative, Incarnational view. Yet it may offer some wonderful surprises for our relationship with God. God is not an angry or vindictive God, demanding the suffering and death of Jesus as payment for past sin. God is, instead, a gracious God, sharing divine life and love in creation and in the Incarnation. Such a view can dramatically change our image of God, our approach to suffering, our day-to-day prayer. This approach is rooted solidly in John's Gospel and in the letters to the Colossians and the Ephesians.

Throughout the centuries great Christian theologians have contributed to this positive perspective on God and Jesus. From the Cappadocian

Fathers in the fourth century (St. Basil, St. Gregory of Nyssa, St. Gregory of Nazianzus) to Franciscan John Duns Scotus in the thirteenth century to Jesuits Teilhard de Chardin and Karl Rahner in the twentieth century, God's gracious love and the primacy of the Incarnation have been proclaimed.[36]

In the late twentieth century, theologian Catherine LaCugna pulled together many of these themes in her book *God for Us*. She uses and expands the Cappadocians' wonderful image of the Trinity as divine dance to include all persons. Borrowing themes of intimacy and communion from John's Gospel and Ephesians, she affirms that humanity has been made a partner in the divine dance not through humanity's own merit but through God's election from all eternity. She writes:

> The God who does not need nor care for the creature, or who is immune to our suffering, does not exist. (. . .) The God who keeps a ledger of our sins and failings, the divine policeman, does not exist. These are all false gods. (. . .) What we believe about God must match what is revealed of God in Scripture: God watches over the widow and the poor, God makes the rains fall on just and unjust alike, God welcomes the stranger and embraces the enemy.[37]

Theologian Edward Schillebeeckx, O.P., has also questioned the traditional interpretation of Jesus' death. In Part Four of his book *Christ*, Schillebeeckx strongly affirms and holds together God's goodness with suffering, both in Jesus' life and in all humans' experience. Schillebeeckx does not try to explain away the reality of suffering and evil in human history, but sees them as rooted in finitude and freedom. Still he stresses that God's mercy is greater, as seen in Jesus' ministry and teaching. God does not want people to suffer but wills to overcome suffering wherever it occurs. Such a God could not require the death of Jesus. Schillebeeckx states:

> *Negativity* cannot have a cause or a motive in God. But in that case we cannot look for a divine *reason* for the death of Jesus either.

---

36. For more on the Cappadocians, see LaCugna, *God for Us*, 53–79 and 270–78; on John Duns Scotus, see Bonaseo, *Man and His Approach*, 44–50; on Teilhard de Chardin, see Mooney, *Teilhard de Chardin*, 133–45; on Karl Rahner, see Rahner, *Foundations*, 178–203, also see Dych, *Karl Rahner*, 65–81.

37. LaCugna, *God for Us*, 397.

Jesus, the Leper, and HIV and AIDS

> Therefore, first of all, we have to say that we are not redeemed *thanks* to the death of Jesus but *despite* it.[38]

Schillebeeckx adds,

> Nor will the Christian blasphemously claim that God himself required the death of Jesus as compensation for what *we* make of our history.[39]

The emphasis on Jesus as God's first thought can free us from violent images of God and allows us to focus on God's overflowing love. This love is the very life of the Trinity and spills over into creation, Incarnation, and the promise of fulfillment of all creation. What a difference this makes for our relationship with God! Life and love, not suffering and death, become the core of our spirituality and morality.

The Abyss of Suffering

But what about the "dark abyss" (Psalm 88) of suffering? The Incarnational approach with its emphasis on God's overflowing love leads us beyond our usual question of "Why?" and suggests three elements of a response to suffering (as exemplified above in "Response of Lament, Action, Trust"): 1) acknowledge the suffering and then lament, 2) act, 3) trust in God.[40] Briefly summarizing here the meaning of these three points emphasizes the implications of "Jesus Is Not Plan B" for our response to suffering.

The first step in responding to suffering is simply being truthful, avoiding denial (which could be so easy) and admitting the pain and horror of the suffering, whatever the cause. We must never glorify suffering. Yes, it can lead us to deeper maturity and wisdom, but suffering can also crush the human spirit. Following the lead of the Psalmist, we can express our pain in lament.

Awareness of suffering and relationship with God allow and inspire our action. We acknowledge that at times our choices have caused personal and social suffering, so one form of action is moving toward repentance and a change of heart. We also suffer from sickness, including HIV and AIDS, and many other personal challenges. In this suffering we need

---

38. Schillebeeckx, *Christ*, 729.
39. Schillebeeckx, *Christ*, 728.
40. For more, see Overberg, *Into the Abyss*, 95–119.

to reach out to others, to ask for help, to receive what they offer, to allow them to accompany us in the dark abyss.

Following the life and ministry of Jesus, we also work as individuals and as communities to overcome and end suffering. Our deeds include remaining with others in their suffering, along with action concerning political and economic issues. We cannot do everything, but we can at least do one thing, as the many examples above indicated.

The third element in our response to suffering, trust in God, is of course especially challenging in the dark times of suffering. Jesus, as we have seen, is a marvelous example of trust in God. His deep, trusting relationship with *Abba* grounded his life and teaching and sustained him in his suffering.

> Are not two sparrows sold for a penny? Yet not one of them will fall to the ground apart from your Father. And even the hairs of your head are all counted. So do not be afraid; you are of more value than many sparrows. (Matt 10:29–31)

Lament and action and trust, however, do not remove the question of suffering. Suffering remains a mystery, not a problem to be solved. We stand with Job at the end of his bold contest with God: "What shall I answer you? I lay my hand on my mouth" (40:4).

The Loving Abyss of God[41]

The emphasis on creation-for-Incarnation, culminating in the resurrection, gives us great hope as we confront the overwhelming suffering of HIV and AIDS. God does not desire suffering but works to overcome it. God did not demand Jesus' suffering and does not want ours. In the context of trusting this gentle God, we lament and act to overcome suffering, even as we acknowledge its incomprehensibility and marvel at God's remarkable respect of human freedom. We know that some suffering results from persons' evil choices (war, injustice, oppression). We know that other suffering simply happens in a world that is not yet fulfilled (earthquakes, debilitating diseases). Suffering, however, is not fully understandable. So, we move past "Why?" to ask instead: "How can I respond? What can we

---

41. Karl Rahner, S.J., speaks of God as Holy Mystery, the Incomprehensible One, a Loving Abyss. See, for example, Rahner, "Why Am I," 8; and especially Rahner, "Thoughts on the Possibility," 8–9.

Jesus, the Leper, and HIV and AIDS

do now?" A profound trust in a compassionate God allows us to ask these questions and then to act, with surprising peace and hope.

Finally, the mystery of God and suffering invites us to prayerful meditation. A suggestion: recall Michelangelo's magnificent sculpture *Pieta*. The grieving mother of Jesus holds his dead body in her arms. Feel the pain, the sorrow, the horror. Then allow the sculpture to become a symbol, to take on even wider meanings. First, perhaps, the symbol of the world's mothers holding their dead sons and daughters, ravaged by AIDS. Then let the sculpture speak of a gentle God holding God's sick and dying world. Finally, let it be God holding your broken spirit.

Our God suffers with us, to use human terms. In the depths of suffering we too may cry out: "My God, my God, why have your forsaken me?" In the darkness, we may need to express our lament, even defiance, but finally our trust that the gracious, gentle God holds our sick and broken bodies and spirits. How could it be otherwise for the God of life and love, the covenanted partner, the tender and gracious parent?

We can trust because there is more: our God is a God of resurrection, of new life. Jesus' story did not end with suffering and death, but with new and transformed life. And Christians are an Easter people. That truth is at the very heart of our response to suffering. God suffers with us, leads us as individuals and as community in resisting evil, and brings us all to the fullness of life.[42]

---

42. This chapter is based on/taken from various sections of my book, Overberg, *Ethics and AIDS*.

4

Women and the Choices They Hold: Hope in the HIV Epidemic

Edwina Ward

"I AM OFTEN ASKED whether there will ever be a cure for HIV and AIDS, and my answer is that there is already a cure." It is still hidden; but, "it lies in the strength of women, families and communities who support and empower each other to break the silence around AIDS and take control of their sexual lives."[1] This powerful statement offers the point of departure for my research, which is based on the concept that women can and must make their own choices to transform and change society in South Africa. This means transforming "power over" to "power with" their partners and with men.

Transformation in attitudes and behavior towards women involves a change from the past to a future of equality and partnership. This demands new thinking, new attitudes, new policies and most of all, women's sense of well-being. It involves an awareness that women are able to work alongside men as equals. All transformation must take place in a woman's own heart, and is expressed in knowing when to turn from the past dominance of men over women.

The power will come when we *stop* and take cognizance of what needs to change, *look* and see clearly where we can make the changes, *listen* to our inner selves and begin with our sense of self-worth to *act* and show the world that we are born equal in God's sight. The women of South Africa have it within themselves to transform their status and so to change society and the evils imposed on them. Women can then take

---

1. Beatrice Were is a Ugandan woman who is convinced that the groups of women who share problems, concerns and status can support one another as they talk openly about AIDS. This in turn will erase the stigma of the disease to some degree, and empower women to take some control over their lives. Epstein, *Invisible Cure*, 167.

Women and the Choices They Hold

their rightful position alongside men in society. This change is not just for the sake of change, but in response to the question, "What is it that women want to change from?" What follows is an outline of areas where change is necessary in order for women and men to grow with regard to certain attributes that contribute to in equality.

The time has come to stop bemoaning the plight of women in our society and to make changes, which will make a difference. The question and the challenge is how to bring about changes in our communities. What are the methods we can use to empower women to keep the interconnectedness of life? When will we support one another with spiritual and emotional leadership and bring about an empowering relationship between home, communities and society as AIDS ravages our lives. The epidemic is ruining families, villages, businesses, and church communities and leaving behind immense distress and sadness, the results of which will be seen in future generations.

We have to understand that anyone can get AIDS and our young people must come to grips with this fact! The availability of antiretrovirals (ARV), of which there are twenty available in the global market but only six in South Africa, does not halt the epidemic on its own. They are not a cure and they are not effective for everyone; they can also have severe side effects. Those who are fortunate enough to receive ARV treatment can only expect to live an extra four or five years longer, because the virus develops resistance and further treatment for that is not yet available in Africa.[2] Anyone who is not infected has to be aware that the HI virus can be contracted whether we are young, old, man, woman, or of any race. Why then is the epidemic so great in South Africa and why is it so difficult to control?

AIDS is a social problem as much as it is a medical problem, and it has spread by a combination of patterns in sexual behavior and poor economy which has left millions of Africans in an unequal global financial squeeze. The poverty and social inequality have caused a wider gap in gender relationships that opens ways for the spread of HIV. It is well known that women are at greatest risk as they have little or no control over their sexual relations.

---

2. "Intensifying," 19.

THE PLIGHT OF WOMEN

In South Africa, the women used to have control over the land, crops, stock and other goods. Then the British replaced this system with the introduction of cash which was controlled by the men. Women lost their autonomy over the household resources. They were soon regarded as bearers of children and workers of the land, expected to feed and clothe the children and keep food on the table. They have experienced a loss of status and are "now treated as donkeys."[3]

Beatings and abuse by men are more frequent and the men never share domestic roles. As women are unable to confront men and take a stand for their rights, they are left at the mercy of angry husbands and of men in general. They are unable to take their troubles to the church, as the church in Africa is by and large narrow in its thinking on sexual matters; and so women are further disempowered and put at greater risk of HIV.

Gender Relations

Gender relations in South Africa are in a bad state. So many of the stories told by women are similar. "He beats me every month, he beat me only yesterday, these are the bruises on my body." So tells Thandi, who goes on to explain, "I received a cell-phone call and my boyfriend accused me of having another boyfriend. I denied it but still he beat me and then forced me to have sex with him."

Rape

Rape is common place in South Africa, which has the highest level of recorded rape in the world. A rape occurs every 82 seconds and is usually committed by men who are known to the girls and women, including their boyfriends or husbands. Most girls are aware that their boyfriends have other girlfriends. It is accepted that men have multiple partners and that the women give in to the sexual demands of these abusive men.

The vast majority of rape victims are not children although this number is rising.[4] The rate of AIDS' increase is attributed to the subordination of women in South African society. Few cases are reported to the

---

3. Kharises, "Effective pastoral care."

4. Scott, "'Alarming' HIV." Age of babies with growing incidences of HIV ranges from 2 to 12 years and there is an increase of widows with HIV who have a mean age of 43 years.

police; and if the rape was committed by a husband or boyfriend, the case is not even considered a crime.

A large proportion of women and men blame women for rape: "Women should dress carefully and behave." Many women have internalized this concept and fear that if their rape becomes known, others will believe that they deserved it. There is also the belief that men are able to discipline their girlfriends if they feel they are "too clever," "too pretty and therefore attracting the admiring glances of other men" or are "too independent."

As we have read in the works of many writers, rape is an assertion of male power, not sexuality.[5] It is speculated that men find acts of violence against women as temporary relief from the humiliation of joblessness, lack of economic power, and lack of respect from fellow men. As South Africa's economy has changed, so have gender norms altered the balance of power between the sexes. In the constitution, gender equality is stressed, and women can graduate from university, find good jobs and move up in the business world, thereby achieving higher status. The epidemic of rape may well be a result of men's perceived loss of status.

Transactional Relationships

In my research I asked some of the younger girls why they put up with men who openly had sex with other women, and some typical response were "Because I love him." "He has a job so he won't ask me for money for beer or cigarettes, and he can help me out with financial problems." "He buys me gifts and make-up and even buys me airtime for my cell phone."

So we can see that a sexual relationship involves a combination of physical attraction and financial calculation. This form of transactional sexual relationship, where women receive gifts of cash or commodities from boyfriends is common among the university students in KwaZulu-Natal.[6] It is not regarded as prostitution, as there are emotional feelings between the partners and they are committed to each other for some length of time.

The women who enter into transactional relationships are more likely to be HIV-positive than other women, even if they have had very

---

5. Brownmiller, *Against Our Will*.
6. Interviews with BTh students at the University of KwaZulu-Natal, Theology Department, 1996 and 1997.

few sexual partners in their young lives. This is because they are tolerant of unfaithful partners and they, themselves, may also have additional concurrent sexual relationships.

One woman explained to me:

> I need different partners at the same time as each one gives me different forms of payment. One gives me money for the cell phone, one gives me food for my family, one buys me nice clothes and another pays the school fees of my younger brother.

There is a great need for luxuries as a form of status among the young women. To be able to go to the shopping centre with a well-dressed man who has his own car is like being acknowledged as a well-born and superior woman in the community. Yet the gifts give men a sense of ownership of a girlfriend's sexuality. Because he is giving her gifts, he feels he also has the right to beat her.

Poverty

People are so poor that sex has become part of their economy. The only way to get commodities or currency is through the sex they have. Women sell their bodies just to get food to eat. AIDS is described as a disease of poverty, yet it can also be recognized as a disease of inequality. The deepening chasm between rich and poor in South Africa is becoming more and more apparent. The poor themselves know that money is at the root of AIDS.[7] So we can see clearly that the social conditions that make people vulnerable to HIV infection must be changed, including poverty, unemployment, and discrimination against women.[8]

Domestic Violence

Domestic violence is commonplace, affecting one in three women. About half of the murders of women are associated with these abusive relationships. Women caught in these relationships are more likely to suffer from depression, miscarriages, and sexually transmitted diseases (STD) and HIV.[9]

---

7. Collins and Rau, *AIDS in the context.*
8. Lamptey, "Reducing heterosexual," 207.
9. Garcia-Moreno et al., "Violence against Women," 1282.

Women and the Choices They Hold

In South Africa, the traditional norms overwhelm sexual relationships. Everything seems to depend on men's ability to control women. Women do most of the agricultural labor, fetch water, find firewood, and care for the children and the sick.[10] Women do not expect to share in the decision-making but are to do the cooking, cleaning, gardening, and rearing of children, while the men involve themselves in having affairs and drinking. Virginity-testing is increasing amongst the Zulu people, indicating that the men feel they are losing control of young people and women. All around them, they see the poor economic and social conditions and the decimation of human life caused by AIDS.

Concurrency

We are still trying to understand why AIDS is so widespread in South Africa, and why it is so difficult to control.

According to research, many South Africans are sexually active at very young ages, even below age fourteen.[11] South Africans are sexually active and very sexually active! These young people were likely to have more than one partner, and were less likely to use condoms. South African girls were likely to face coercion or rape, or to exchange money for sex. We have to challenge ourselves, the churches and the government to find an effective way to get the message about HIV and AIDS across to these young people. They know about AIDS but don't internalize that knowledge. Today there is relative freedom among African women who have been educated. Yet this does not seem to stop the number of casual partners that women have.

A professor of sociology at the University of Washington, Martina Morris, developed a model for predicting the spread of HIV amongst the Ugandan population. She discovered that some men and women had ongoing relationships with two or three persons at one time. These concurrent relationships may overlap for months or as long as a year. This behavior was normal in the African community, as can be seen through the tradition of polygamy. Men have traditionally counted their wealth in people. The wives could work on the land and also produce children, who later could form alliances with other tribes. Control over women was of great value and a measure of a man's wealth along with his cattle. The

---

10. Jewkes, "Non-consensual."
11. Rehle, Thomas et al., "National HIV," 194–99.

more women a man had, the greater his status in society, the more he was respected within his community.

But these

> concurrent or simultaneous sexual partnerships are far more dangerous than serial monogamy, because they link people up in a giant web of sexual relationships that creates ideal conditions for the rapid spread of HIV.[12]

Morris found that the average African had fewer sexual partners over a lifetime than the average American. The key difference is that the Americans have several long-term relationships over a lifetime that are sequentially but not concurrent. In Uganda, Morris found that at least two of a man's most recent relationships overlapped for several months or years. Men with only one wife had mistresses or girlfriends with whom they slept at closely spaced intervals, on a "rota basis."[13]

This helps to explain why, in Africa, many women who are faithful are infected with HIV, even though they themselves are not involved in concurrent sexual relationships. It is the behavior of their husbands that puts them at risk. To clarify: If a man with two long-term partners contracts HIV and perhaps then has a one-night stand with a prostitute, he will probably pass on the virus to both of his partners. Now, if either partner has another partner, he or she will soon be infected, along with any other partners that he or she may have; and so it continues.

Thus, it is not only the number of sex partners that counts, but whether those partners are part of a larger sexual network involving long-term concurrent relationships. Because long-term relationships usually involve intimacy and trust, condoms are seldom used, which makes the epidemic more difficult to control.

It also turns out that HIV-positive people are much more likely to pass on the virus in the first few weeks or months after they have been infected themselves. At this stage, it is seldom that the infected persons have been tested or even thought that they should seek voluntary counseling and testing. Christopher D. Pilcher from Duke-UNC Emory Acute HIV Consortium stated in 2004 that a

---

12. Morris and Kretzschmar. "A Microsimulation."
13. Morris, *AIDS in Uganda*.

recently infected person may be a hundred or even a thousand times more likely to transmit the virus than someone who has been infected for a few months or years.[14]

We can also take the example of miners at the gold, diamond or coal mines in South Africa. Many of the miners have more than one long-term partner, a wife or a girlfriend back home and another partner in the township, and are caught up in a concurrency network. This places them in a high-risk category and increases the risk of their passing the virus onto others.

Partner Reduction

After the drop in HIV and AIDS infections in Uganda, it was found that many people were protecting themselves from HIV by reducing their partners or staying with only one.

In fact it was reported in Uganda that when large numbers of people reduce their partners all at once, it can stop the virus in its tracks. This partner reduction may even improve gender relations since there would tend to be fewer accusations of infidelity, and thus domestic violence could also diminish.

WAYS IN WHICH WOMEN CAN BE OFFERED CHOICES

There is hope for women in leadership, especially in the broad fields of education, teaching of human rights and "care economy." The care economy would include communities assisting women with their workloads; providing cooperative daycare centers, nutrition, skills-training, educational assistance for orphans, home care for People Living with HIV and AIDS (PLWHA), as well as labor-sharing and income-generating projects. This new vision for women includes not only intellectual knowledge; it also means instilling a deep set of values that call for attitudinal change.

Home-based Care

A central focus of AIDS organizations in South Africa is that of home-based care. The community members volunteer to help families who are caring for their loved ones. In many respects this is the true value of

---

14. Pilcher, et al., "Brief but efficient."

ubuntu. This word means that we share the meaning of life as humanity. "A person is a person through other people," is the rough translation.

Our society is like a wheel and if one of the spokes is broken, the wheel risks being destroyed. *Ubuntu* implies that we have obligations and responsibilities that control our individualistic behaviors and impel us to work for the common good. There are groups in KwaZulu-Natal in the Osindisweni district, north of Durban, who go out each day, collect water, sweep someone's house, take care of the children, and plant some seeds for the family. Women I have talked to say this does not take money, only a caring heart. Many times these women are there just to talk to the sick person and pray with them.

In the Communicable Diseases Clinic (CDC) at Grey's Hospital in Pietermaritzburg the patients meet daily for counseling, and they share their stories with each other. Gradually, as one of the chaplain-counselors became more trusted, she was invited to join these groups and I went with her.

What these people shared, as to how they were feeling about their illness, was at first hesitant and stumbling. Gradually, over three weeks, the participants in the group were openly trusting each other and telling their stories. They spoke of beatings, abuse, husbands who had many partners, fear of having no income, being scared of the future for their children, and their loss of self-worth and dignity.

In other words, they spoke of the need to rebuild their self-esteem, to help women and men accept their HIV-status and learn to live with it. Life has not ended when a person becomes HIV-positive. The support of the group, the open discussions, the passing on of their stories to others who are not infected, all play a major role in the control women can take over their own lives.

After one meeting, both women and men in the group decided to take a stance on the behaviors of their partners. They decided that, until the following week, if they learned of their partners sleeping with any other person, or if their partners did not come home for the night, they would dare to refuse to have sex with them. As they stood together in solidarity, there seemed to be group strength, group caring and community resolve. This is a powerful message of *ubuntu*—we stand together.

Home-based care groups are getting into the homes of those who are ill, and now the nursing and social services are able to use them as 'associates' to help with medication, reminders to attend clinics and see that patients are getting correct nutrition where possible.

Media

Women and men today can equally work as leaders of worship and prayer, offer themselves to care for the house-bound and aged, work in prisons, preach the word of God, and rally the community to become a 'care-support community' to the orphans, widows, bereaved and single parents.

I do not believe we have fully explored the use of media, especially the radio. There is hardly a family in urban or rural areas in South Africa who do not possess a radio. A huge and concerted effort to educate, to destigmatize HIV and AIDS and to offer solutions lies in this medium of communication. Women radio hosts speaking to women, and respected women in powerful positions speaking to men and women, can bring about a collegiality and a working together for our mutual concerns.

There have been large advertising campaigns and programs, some of which have been very successful and some of which have sadly been withdrawn due to overseas funding being stopped. To name a few: LoveLife's media campaign which shows a positive lifestyle for young people to live by. Another is the work done by the Y-Centers, where youth are offered training in computer skills, cooking, literacy, and communication skills. There is the St. Charles Lwanga Catholic organization that carries out a number of activities in the townships. If one searches the Internet, more programs can be found and they have all had some effectiveness within the general population.

Besides using ads on billboard and on radio and television, there is still a need for serious education and knowledge to be passed on in schools, church groups, places of public education, books, and documentaries. These programs need experts who explain that there is a need for change in the understanding of the African epidemic.

People need to talk more openly about AIDS and HIV, and to be given the opportunity to look at their own behavior and beliefs. They can work together to change the things that need to be changed in their local communities. We must continue with the use of counseling, testing, use of condoms, and bring to awareness the successes of circumcision as a way of preventing transmission of the virus.

It turns out that male circumcision is highly protective against HIV.[15] Two tribes in South Africa with very high infection rates are the Zulu and the Tswana. In 2006, researchers in South Africa and Uganda found that circumcision cuts a man's risk of contracting HIV by a huge margin of fifty percent. Male circumcision may also protect women too.[16]

Women could be encouraged to continue with community-based initiatives, such as home-based care programs, orphan centers, and support groups for people who are HIV-positive and their families. There is a great need for women's rights groups, and for opportunities for women to get micro-financing, which in turn must be controlled. This way, the funding gets to the needy directly.

The insecurity of living in a rapidly globalizing world is having an effect on patterns of sexual networking. There is a need for medical and pharmaceutical companies to take another look at the quality of condoms, the costs of antiretroviral treatment and the development of microbicides. As yet, microbicides are unavailable and are currently thought to be less effective than first believed. Women will have to be able to afford them, and learn to use them correctly and consistently. At this stage, they are considered to be less effective than condoms.

HIV Testing

HIV testing is another way forward. Once a person is found to be negative, the great advantages of staying that way should be thoroughly explained to them. Knowledge is the most powerful tool we have. However, there is little evidence that widespread testing is sufficient for HIV prevention. Sadly, there is no evidence that HIV testing changes the behavior of those who find they are negative. They still engage in risky behavior.

In some areas of KwaZulu-Natal, a nurse with a vehicle goes from door to door to test. Many people run away form the testing, especially women. This is for fear of the blame they will receive from boyfriends and husbands if they are found out. Some poor women are blamed for bringing the infection into the relationships, and others are beaten and cast out of their homes. Over forty percent are too afraid to tell their partners about the testing.

---

15. Auvert et al., "Randomised."
16. Auvert et al., "Randomised."

Women and the Choices They Hold

It is recognized that South African people have a right to know their HIV status, and HIV testing services are important; but they only work if they are voluntary. This is where there is a need for clever advertising campaigns to destigmatize HIV and protect the rights of women.

The ARV treatment programs also have limitations.[17] ARV drugs may add to the life expectancy of an AIDS patient, but in South Africa the chances of that happening are less obvious. It is now estimated that, on average, only another four or five years may be added because the HIV becomes resistant; eventually the patient must be given another "cocktail" to which the virus soon becomes resistant, as well. AIDS patients need counseling and ongoing care to treat opportunistic infections and to monitor drug resistance and side effects. According to Stephen Carpenter, ARV treatment programs are unlikely to control the epidemic unless they are accompanied by other prevention efforts.[18]

Connectedness

Writers such as developmental personality theorist, Erik Erikson,[19] feminist writers Mary Daly[20] and Bell Hooks,[21] and scripture scholars such as Sandra Schneiders[22] offer us an understanding of a woman's need for connectedness. In her well-received book, *In a Different Voice*, Carol Gilligan observes that:

> [T]he danger men describe in their stories of intimacy is a danger of entrapment or betrayal, being caught in a smothering relationship or humiliated by rejection or deceit. In contrast, the danger women portray in their tales of achievement is a danger of isolation, a fear that in standing out or being set apart by success, they will be left alone.[23]

Gilligan goes on to state that "while men perceive danger in connection, women experience danger in separation."[24] By observing this, Gilligan

---

17. Carpenter, "What perceived benefits."
18. Carpenter, "What perceived benefits."
19. Erikson, *Childhood and Society*.
20. Daly, *Beyond God the Father*.
21. Hooks, *Black Looks*.
22. Schneiders, *New Wineskins*.
23. Gilligan, *In a Different Voice*.
24. Gilligan, *In a Different Voice*, 42.

argues that identity and intimacy are inseparable for women. Erikson however, believes that the tensions lie in the polarities of initiative and guilt, between identity and role diffusion and between intimacy and isolation.[25]

It is my conviction that women move within the realm that arises from the tension between initiative and identity and, through discovery of their roles, offer an intimacy which becomes part of their expression of equality. This sequence of development takes place to alleviate their fear of isolation. It would seem that our role models of the past have encouraged men to seek separation from those they lead, for fear of losing their individuality and power. They may have been taught by early role models to become leaders who are suspicious of their followers for fear of betrayal.

Women on the other hand have been led to believe that they need to belong to the groups they lead and do not want to be seen as apart from them. If both men and women could restructure these tendencies, they would come to accept that leadership in ministry will be enhanced through collaboration, and that such a partnership would benefit those whom they serve.

Practical Steps for Women to Exercise Their Choices and Overcome the Grip That HIV and AIDS Has on Them

There is a need for more practical steps to be taken in prevention programs that would respond to young peoples real circumstances in life. Such measures would have to be more honest about the real human consequences of the disease. But that would need to address some very difficult consequences of current HIV policy in the South Africa.

The problem with the large foreign-aid programs was distribution of the funding. These large sums of money are not easy to manage and the small community-based groups, which only need thousands and not millions, are overlooked. Megaprojects are not always clear in their goals or final outcomes. Some of the money that arrives in South Africa is well spent, but some is wasted on poorly conceived projects which sound good to the foreign donors, but which make little sense within the African reality. So much of the money does not reach the people who need it the most, and just makes the donors feel good about themselves.

---

25. Erikson, *Identity.*

Women and the Choices They Hold

Sizanani and HOPE which is one of the largest non-governmental organizations (NGOs) working on AIDS in South Africa, have been providing home-based care, medicines and teaching of HIV prevention for over ten years. Sizanani, a drop-in centre, has provided food, counseling, care for orphans and a play school for children along with meals. In fact Sizanani can be grouped along with the very few orphanages in South Africa. What is needed is to provide basic social services to AIDS affected children. There is a need to set up a bereavement-counseling curriculum and for the wonderful effects of "Memory Work" to be more deeply valued throughout South Africa.[26]

THE CHOICES WOMEN HOLD

Women are able to take charge of their lives through the support they offer one another through active home-based care groups that demonstrate the strength of *ubuntu* and communal caring. This value in life offers strength, communication, love and compassion, and eases the burden of the loss of dignity caused by the debilitating illness of AIDS.

The use of the media should be further exploited through advertising and the extensive use of the radio. Women presenters could run programs designed to talk to the listeners, tell them about their rights, and encourage them to take control of their lives and their relationships. Radio talk shows and phone-ins offer a platform for the lonely voice of women to be heard. At the same time, the male radio audience would learn of the needs and the determination of women to rise above the accepted norms of inequality. Women could inform one another of new ways to earn money, to become leaders of today's youth and to take control over their sex lives.

Through the media, clinics, and ongoing education, men could be encouraged to be circumcised. Talk of condoms and microbicides could become open in the family and in the education system, and information about HIV testing could be disseminated by the same means. This kind of communication would lead to the breakdown of stigmatization and discrimination. More knowledge and acknowledgement of HIV and AIDS, and more openness in conversations will eventually give women the power to take a stand over their position in society.

---

26. The Memory Box Project in KwaZulu-Natal is run by Professor Philippe Denis of the School of Religion and Theology at the University of KwaZulu-Natal.

A program such as Intervention with Microfinance for AIDS and Gender Equity (IMAGE) could be initiated. This program gives women a new language. Its strength derives less from individual personal empowerment than from the collective social energy it engenders. IMAGE brings women together to solve common problems that none could solve on their own. Women are encouraged to speak openly about women's rights, not only in workshops and seminars, but also among themselves, before their church congregations, in the schools and in the gathering places of shopping centers.

IMAGE is there to offer women small loans with which to begin projects to earn more money and so to continue the cycle. A woman I spoke to was loaned 300 rands to begin her project. She bought an old sewing machine and pieces of cloth. With this she made clothes for small children in her village and charged a minimal price. After half a year, she was making 500 rands per month for her family.

Before the loan, she had known humiliation, born a sense of worthlessness and a feeling of powerlessness. She had to beg for food from her neighbors and her children were unable to go to school. Now her husband valued her contributions to the household and treated her with more respect, as did her community.

This micro-financing from the Small Enterprise Foundation (SEF) was the beginning of a new life for over forty women who were given these small loans. Admittedly, there will be failures and some women will either misuse the money or businesses will fail. But for those who are successful, the future will become brighter. IMAGE has offered women not only the chance to gain self-respect, but in their meetings they have been able to share in open-ended discussions about sexuality, relationships and the very difficult roles that women have to play in today's society. The culture of denial and silence has been overturned and the level of domestic abuse has diminished.

Finally, understanding the dangers of concurrent relationships, where women and men have ongoing partnerships with two or three persons at a time, and the benefits of reducing in number of partners or staying with only one, would not only improve gender relations and thus lower the incidence of domestic violence, but would stop the virus from spreading immediately.

Women and the Choices They Hold

From the foregoing discussion, it would appear that there are ways to provide women with positive choices, whether it be through communal sharing, open discussions, micro-financing, better use of the media, caring for one another, or a new understanding of the need for the reduction in partners. Whatever gives women the power to make choices and to break the silence around HIV and AIDS will give them control over their sexual lives and enough equality to transform their partners' "power over" them to a mutually beneficial "power with" their partners.

5

A Pastoral Letter from the Bishops of the Church of Sweden about HIV from a Global Perspective

PREFACE

Since the first person in Sweden was diagnosed with AIDS in the early 1980s, the Church of Sweden has adopted the same position on AIDS and HIV[1] as on other life-threatening illnesses. We are ready to provide pastoral care to those individuals affected, but the Church has not publicly positioned itself on issues surrounding HIV. With few exceptions, the same silence has been notable throughout Swedish society.

We, the Bishops of the Church of Sweden, wish to make our views known on HIV. We do so based on the experience gained by the Church of Sweden in its work with HIV-infected persons, and based on the experiences shared with us by other churches. We have noted that, even as the epidemic continues to grow, HIV issues receive less attention than they used to. Our intervention is now timely.

The Church of Sweden has had workers stationed in various parts of the world for more than a hundred years, and during that time our awareness that events outside our country's borders also affect us has deepened. We have learned, not least through these workers, just how devastating HIV is, not only for the individual, but also for the whole of society and for the churches.

This *Pastoral Letter* is addressed to the members and workers of the Church of Sweden and to everyone who works with us for a good society where the value of every individual is respected. We especially address those who have particular social responsibilities in our own country, in

---

1. HIV is an abbreviation of Human Immunodeficiency Virus. AIDS is an abbreviation of Acquired Immunodeficiency Syndrome.

A Pastoral Letter from the Bishops of the Church of Sweden

other countries, and in international cooperation. In the public sector, we address those responsible for care or humanitarian aid; in the private sector, we address those who represent the pharmaceutical industry. We also address this *Pastoral Letter* to the parishes and leaders of the world's churches.

Our *Pastoral Letter* has three parts. The first part gives a picture of the HIV situation at the current time. We point out that HIV is a structural problem that affects already vulnerable groups particularly hard. We highlight value-related issues as a global problem, and we focus on the role of churches. The second part elaborates on the theological and ethical background to our assessment of the situation and takes account of the HIV experience gained by the Church of Sweden in its pastoral care. The third part presents our conclusions and recommendations.

Uppsala, Sweden, November 2007
For the Bishops' Conference, Anders Wejryd, Archbishop

Vulnerability, Churches, and HIV

HIV—A STATUS REPORT

> With the coming of HIV and AIDS people are starting to realize the injustices that have been there. Even injustices that have not been mentioned for many, many centuries now they are out in the light. Things that were accepted, now in the face of HIV and AIDS they make women more vulnerable.
>
> People that are living with HIV are part of the solution and not a problem. They should be involved in decision making and given support that is needed and allowed to live their lives as normally as they can.
>
> —Annie Kaseketi
> Zambia
> pastor and member of ANERELA+[2]

A Structural Problem

HIV was identified in the early 1980s in the USA, but is thought to have spread around the world after its origin in Africa decades earlier. With almost two thirds of the world's infected, including two million children, sub-Saharan Africa remains the worst affected region. An estimated 12 million children have lost their parents to AIDS. There is no sign that the epidemic is abating.[3]

The spread of HIV varies considerably between continents and countries (see figure 1). The increase in the number of HIV-infected in East Asia, South America and, not least, the Baltic states and several Central Asian countries is alarming.

During the time that the virus has spread, UNAIDS has calculated that around 25 million people have died of AIDS. Statistics from 2007 indicate that there are almost 33.2 million HIV-infected worldwide, of whom about 2.5 million were diagnosed. That same year, 2.1 million people died as a consequence of the disease. However, the mortality rate from AIDS varies in different parts of the world. The number of HIV-infected in Western and Central Europe and in North America was put at 2.1 million, but access to better treatment meant that only around 32,000

---

2. African Network of Religious Leaders Living with or Personally Affected by HIV & AIDS.

3. The statistical data in this text is taken from UNAIDS reports.

people died of AIDS in these countries. In Sweden, it is thought that today around 4,000 people are living with HIV.[4]

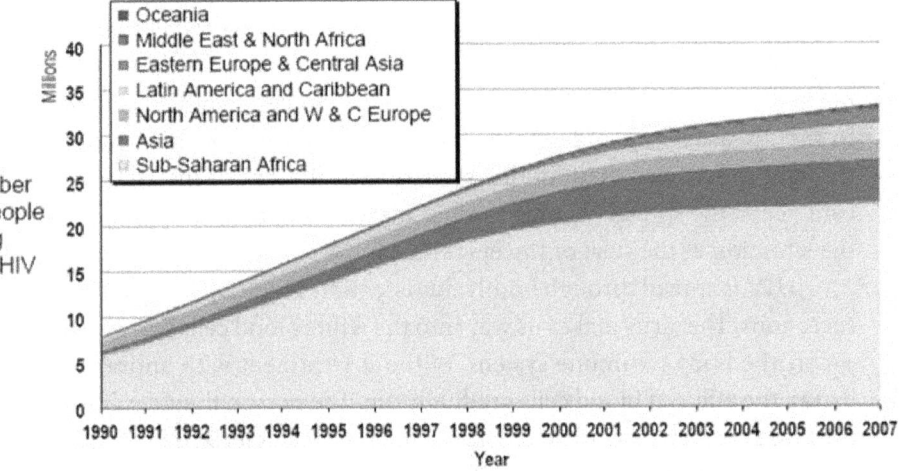

Figure 1. Number of people living with HIV in different parts of the world. Annual figures 1987–2007. Source: UNAIDS.

This summary confirms that HIV is spreading fastest among those whose situation is already the most difficult. Being born in the "wrong" country is clearly a health risk. Despite a large number of deaths in Africa, research to identify the virus was only funded when AIDS started affecting people in the USA and Europe in the early 1980s. HIV is thus one of the social, economic and cultural factors that affect people's living conditions globally.

Even within various countries, the spread of HIV reflects the injustices in the society. The disease primarily affects those who are already vulnerable. This has fuelled the public image of HIV and AIDS as self-inflicted and, above all, as something that affects "the Other." In the early years, HIV and AIDS were depicted as something that affected certain high-risk groups, particularly men having sex with men, sex workers and drug users. One of the painful facts about HIV in our own country is

---

4. Data from the Swedish Institute for Infectious Disease Control.

that the virus was only taken seriously when it became known that it also reached into traditional nuclear families.

In our country, increased knowledge, more effective infection control, and, in particular, good access to antiretroviral treatment (ART), have led to the situation being viewed as less alarming today than 20 or 25 years ago. The fact that a large proportion of those found to be HIV positive were infected before immigration to Sweden may also contribute to the disease still being seen as affecting "the Other." Such attitudes are thought to have led to an underestimation of the risk of infection. In recent years, the spread of infection has increased to a level reminiscent of the situation at the start of the epidemic.

HIV is spread through bodily fluids, chiefly blood, sperm and vaginal secretions. The virus makes its way into the white blood cells that normally excert the body's immune system. Without treatment with antiretroviral drugs, the affected blood cells gradually die. The person then develops the immune deficiency syndrome AIDS, which is characterized by infections that are normally combated by a functioning immune system. Eventually, these infections have a terminal outcome.

It has not yet been possible to produce a vaccine against HIV, but research continues. ART limits the ability of the virus to spread in the body and thus limits the risk of the infected person developing AIDS. ART can restore the immune system, but the underlying HIV infection always remains. Proper medication gradually leads to the infected person becoming symptom-free, and to an undetectable viral load. At this point, the risk of infecting someone else is practically non-existent, but the infection lies dormant and the virus reappears if medication is stopped. For economic and infrastructural reasons, the population in many low-income countries does not currently have access to anti-retroviral treatment.

Infection is prevented primarily by practicing safe sex, including the use of a condom during sexual intercourse. The most common route of infection is through unprotected sex, but the virus can also be transmitted from mother to child during pregnancy, at birth or through breastfeeding.

Time and again, established hierarchical structures between the sexes put women at a disadvantage. The number of women infected with HIV is increasing in comparison with the number of men infected. This is at least in part due to the fact that, in practice, women in many countries have no control over their own sexuality. In some countries, married women run a greater risk of becoming infected than unmarried women, since they cannot refuse to have intercourse or require their partners to use a condom. In addition, some women are forced into selling sexual services to provide for themselves and their families, putting themselves at great risk because their male customers are unwilling to use condoms.

Since the risks of HIV infection became known, infection through blood transfusion has rarely occurred in the Western world. However, in countries without the resources to ensure that blood from infected people is not used, blood transfusions do put people at risk.

A significant route of infection is intravenous drug use, when several people use the same needle. Drugs and poverty are often interlinked. Drug use in itself is always a tragedy, and widespread drug use bears witness to a society in which people lack constructive opportunities to overcome their sense of powerlessness, marginalization and misery. Marginalization is often bound up with exclusion for other reasons, and this is strengthened through drug use. It is, for instance, not uncommon for people with poor mental health to use drugs to alleviate both their mental problems and the hopelessness they experience. The spread of infection in a society increases with growing drug problems; this is particularly apparent in Eastern Europe today.

HIV is currently the most serious challenge in all development work. It is impossible to fight poverty unless the issue of HIV is tackled at the same time. Nor is it possible, in the long term, to handle the HIV epidemic without addressing the problem of poverty. The destructive effects of poverty and HIV reinforce one another. HIV is not just a problem for individuals; it is a structural problem at societal and global levels.

Poverty means poorer healthcare and poorer education. Many of those who live with HIV in materially poor countries are unaware of their situation and have never had the opportunity to take an HIV test. Others avoid being tested for fear of discrimination. However, where there has been access to testing, HIV medication and support groups, discrimination has been reduced and openness surrounding HIV has increased.

Few people living with HIV today have access to ART. The scope for greater investment in medication in low-income countries is limited by the costs and is made more difficult by international patent and trade regulations. The World Trade Organization (WTO) agreement regulating patent rights, known as the TRIPS Agreement (Trade-Related Aspects of Intellectual Property Rights), permits the import or manufacture of cheap pharmaceutical copies, or generic pharmaceuticals, where this is justified with regard to the public health interests of the country. Despite this possibility, many practical obstacles remain when, in line with this agreement, low-income countries try to take measures to increase access to medication.

A particular problem is the increasing number of children infected with HIV. There has not yet been any conclusive research into the correct doses for children and, above all, there are only a few, expensive, types of medication suitable for children.

Many materially poor countries lack adequate numbers of trained healthcare professionals. Active recruitment by rich countries of such professionals from low-income countries has a serious impact on the ability of low-income countries to treat HIV and operate functional healthcare systems.

Poverty cannot be successfully eradicated without the cooperation of the rich countries of the world. A small proportion of its population consumes the vast majority of the earth's resources. This imbalance is costing millions of people their lives.

Despite the lower number of people infected with HIV and better access to treatment, the risk—and dread—of discrimination is a real problem for those who are HIV-infected in Sweden. Ignorance about HIV is widespread and causes significant problems. Not even within the health service, where knowledge and empathy should be at their greatest, can every HIV-infected person be confident of being treated professionally and respectfully.

A particular problem arises when HIV-infected asylum seekers are deported from the country. While they are in Sweden, they have access to vital medication, but this access ceases upon deportation. This clearly shows that HIV raises issues that can only be solved through international cooperation.

An Attitude Problem

It is not only the illness itself that makes life difficult for those infected; other people's ignorance and fear are important parts of the problem. Public information initiatives, although they are necessary, can never completely eradicate these. What people only read or hear about in the media and other public contexts can be kept at a remove and the unknown is more frightening when experienced solely at a distance. Only when people are actually confronted with what they fear, can they deal with it in a constructive way.

People who are informed that they have a life-threatening illness are forced to re-evaluate their lives, but in most cases they have the support and sympathy of those around them. To avoid discrimination, many people with an HIV infection choose to keep quiet about their disease. They dare not be open about what, for them, is a question of life and death and, thus, perpetuate a state of exclusion and perceived lack of dignity.

Often the most difficult thing to deal with is the sense of shame and guilt. HIV, more than other life-threatening illnesses, is seen as self-inflicted through morally reprehensible behavior. This is, to a large degree, bound up with the fact that HIV is sexually transmitted. A similar level of shame is attached to other sexually transmitted diseases. To the extent that other chronic and life-threatening illnesses can be considered self-inflicted, for example, as a consequence of smoking or overeating, they are seen as tragic, but are not stigmatized to anywhere near the same extent.

Denial and silence are the virus's most powerful allies. This is true in all contexts, from the individual to the global. Many people die without ever having told anyone about their condition. Knowledge about the disease and the spread of infection that could change this situation is not getting through. It is essential for the future that the silence is broken, so that vital knowledge can be disseminated and the virus halted. This applies both in countries with large numbers of people who are HIV-infected and in our part of the world, where the virus appears to have practically disappeared from public consciousness.

People infected with HIV are brought up with the same values as those around them. When the person who *becomes* infected has already learned to despise those who *are* infected, he or she will direct that contempt towards themselves, often more mercilessly than anyone else. From an existential point of view, this is the most destructive aspect of the lives of the HIV infected. By not telling anyone, it may be possible to avoid the judgment of others, but one can never escape one's own self-judgment. If one also believes that God is on the side of those judging, then there is no escape in life or in death.

There is, therefore, a great risk that the person infected will be unable to accept this realization and so will remain in a state of denial that is a natural reaction to any crisis. Naturally, such denial can have devastating consequences for a partner, or partners; it also deters the infected from dealing with the situation and finding constructive ways forward.

The need for conversational support, respectful listening, empathy, pastoral care and human intimacy is as great as the need for medication, and this need is just as great for those who have and for those who do not have access to medication. Medication can prolong life, but does not necessarily make it meaningful. A meaningful life requires a restoration of humanity. This occurs in the meeting of people with people and the meeting of people with God. The restoration of humanity would be supported if the issue of HIV as a question of the value and dignity of every individual were moved up the public agenda.

Churches as Part of Both the Problem and the Solution

Part of the problem is the inability of churches to handle issues of sexual ethics. Churches' silence or ill-advised recommendations have contributed to the ongoing spread of the epidemic. At the same time, churches have been instrumental in providing information and recommendations that have resulted in effective prevention; they have also combated marginalization and stigmatization. The role of churches in HIV response relates not least to the issue of values. This is also the case within the churches, which, in many countries, have kept resolutely quiet about the existence of HIV—also among the churches' members and leaders.

Health institutions run by churches have offered treatment to HIV victims for a long time and taken important social initiatives, often long before other players started their work. Today, churches are still responsible for a large proportion of the work carried out at hospitals, within various programmes for Home Based Care and within social initiatives, despite receiving a very small share of the resources allocated through international funds for HIV work.

Over the years, it has been easier for churches to accept that HIV is a problem in society than to accept that HIV is also spreading amongst church members. Through the metaphor "The Body of Christ has HIV," churches are seeking, in a partnership between north and south, to break the silence and remind each other that HIV affects us all—that it is a matter of concern for the whole of the worldwide Church and all its members.

A Pastoral Letter from the Bishops of the Church of Sweden

The phrase "Body of Christ" alludes to churches as organisms, as something more than just an organization, and the churches' members are described as the limbs of one body—even if they are infected with HIV. The declaration that "the Body of Christ has HIV," therefore, highlights the need for a conscious solidarity. Churches with large resources have a clear responsibility to listen to those who are infected and to speak for those who have been silenced.

This applies to the relations between different churches as well as to relations between people in our Swedish parishes. Unless parishes can offer a safe and welcoming environment where those who live with HIV can dare to be themselves, declarations of solidarity with HIV-infected around the world are empty words.

A church that seeks to be the body of Christ in the world must lift its gaze and look outside its own inner circle. Christ has told us where he wants to meet us and where he wants to lead us: "Truly I tell you, just as you did it to one of the least of these who are members of my family, you did it to me" (Matt 25:40). In the reversed perspective of the Kingdom of God, all social conventions are challenged: the greatest become the least and the least the greatest and in the greatest suffering the glory of God is shown most clearly.

In this context, people may want to consider the double meaning of the word "stigmatization." The original meaning of the Greek work *stigma* is "a brand or puncture wound," and it is usually used to signify the "branding" of groups seen as being of less value than others. However, particularly in its plural form *stigmata*, in religious terminology the word has denoted Jesus' wounds. These are two different meanings which should not be confused, but which can be combined in a deeper interpretation: in the experience of those stigmatized, the churches recognize the suffering that Jesus Christ took upon himself out of love for all humanity, and that he calls us to share.

Vulnerability, Churches, and HIV

Theological, Ethical and Pastoral Perspectives on HIV

> We were born to make manifest the glory of God that is within us. It's not just in some of us; it's in everyone.
>
> —Nelson Mandela

A Christian View of Humanity

To talk about "vulnerable groups" or about how HIV is more likely to affect "those whose situation is already difficult" in itself runs the risk of reinforcing unequal structures. Our intention in describing the situation is to emphasize where the needs are greatest and which circumstances particularly demand our attention. The analysis fails its purpose if the consequence is that certain people or groups are perceived as helpless in relation to others and dependent upon the benevolence of others. It is far too easy to take the patterns of power and marginalization that we see around us as given, and—perhaps with the best of intentions—to become locked in roles and expectations that perpetuate these patterns.

To find ways to achieve constructive change, we need to be able to relate every given situation to a view of humanity that champions the fundamental value and dignity of all people. With such a view of humanity, we can provide a perspective on what it is to be human and sharpen our focus on actual reality.

A Christian view of humanity takes as its starting point a view of the world as created by God, who is love. The Bible speaks of the world as created by God at the beginning of time, but also about how God constantly renews our world with his Spirit. Creation is not a distant, isolated, single event. God is always with us, and this world that we live in is in a state of constant change and renewal.

At the core of the Christian view on humanity is the idea, expressed in the Bible, that mankind is created in God's image. This likeness to God means that each and every one of us has a role to play in God's ongoing creation. As humans, we can share God's love for the world and strive to make sure that the resources available to us are used to manifest God's love. We have a responsibility to maintain good relations in the world through a wholehearted commitment to life and peace, justice and sustainable development. In so doing, we constantly face new challenges and new opportunities.

Our dignity as people is thus closely linked to our ability to live in responsibility and love. However, our human reality also includes the experience of vulnerability and imperfection, disappointment and unavoidable guilt. We constantly long for a life that is completely and utterly genuine, but over and over again we are forced to accept that we are not able to live up to our own ideals. The more clearly we see how life should be, the more aware we become of our own powerlessness.

In church terminology, our inability to live in love and responsibility is expressed in terms of sin. The Bible's story of the Creation is immediately followed by a story of human shortcoming. Like the story of Creation, it depicts an eternally ongoing process, but one where we as humanity are tempted to approach life and the world in a destructive way.

In the Bible's depiction of Jesus, we recognize a life that is complete and true, filled with love and care—but that also challenges all destruction, small-mindedness and self-absorbedness. As Christians, we also see God himself in Jesus. At our side, God in Jesus' person bears all the guilt that is ours, shares our weakness and dies our death. But more than that: Jesus goes before us into death and through the Resurrection he explodes the boundary that we thought was the definitive end of all things and paves the way to a new life.

Three HIV-related Issues

In this overarching perspective, the Church must interpret the questions that face us in the meeting with HIV.

Firstly, since the disease is chiefly spread through sexual relations, we must address *issues of the body and sexuality*. Our bodies are an indispensable part of our individual and social identity. All our relations are, in some respect, physical. We cannot live a life of love and responsibility without this also including our bodies.

As such, we have an obligation to treat our lives with care and intelligence, not hurting others but also not hurting ourselves or foolishly exposing ourselves to danger. Self-destructive behavior bears witness to broken relationships with other people, with one's own life and with God, who loves us and wishes us well. Abuse of drugs or sexual relations, is evidence that people lack the fundamental security that everyone needs in life. When such a situation is used and exploited commercially, people are systematically stripped of their most fundamental human dignity.

Sexuality was given to us in creation as God's way of constantly creating new life. Sexuality is necessary for humanity's continuation and a source of togetherness, joy and deeper love and intimacy. The sexual relationship is an expression of every person's need to relate to another person with their entire being: it is life-giving in many respects.

It is deeply tragic that a life-threatening disease such as HIV is spread through sexual relations. However, that fact adds another dimension to the responsibility that we all bear for how we deal with our sexuality and our sexual relations. Fundamental in this context—as in others—are values such as love, reciprocity, trust, and equality. Trust and reciprocity are constantly put to the test in our sexual relations, which is particularly clear in situations that in various ways are marked by insecurity and marginalization. Perceived lack of power can make it difficult to recognize one's responsibility as a person. The scope for making responsible choices can, in practice, be extremely limited for those who live in vulnerable situations. Work to combat HIV is, therefore, largely an issue of increasing people's scope for self-determination over their lives and their bodies.

Secondly, HIV also raises *issues of solidarity and equality*, not least in terms of superiority and inferiority between the sexes. According to a Christian view of humanity, everyone—man as well as woman—is made in God's image and those who harm their fellow people deface God's image.

This also applies to the relationship between the rich and poor of the world. We have been entrusted with the world so that we may look after it in the best interests of everyone, as is God's will. From this perspective, the fact that a small part of humanity grows rich at the expense of others is indefensible. The God who created the world is a God for all people, and particularly for those who in people's eyes are poor and vulnerable.

A responsible and loving attitude in the face of the inequality that we encounter, and that we ourselves are always a part of, demands that we strive with all the means at our disposal to restore people's dignity. It is a case of combating abuse of power and marginalization in all its forms, and the despondency born of a sense of powerlessness.

Thirdly, our HIV brings us to pose the question *what makes a meaningful life*? Every person's life is unique and meaningful because it is created by God. When we seek to deal with everything that happens to us and everything that we face with trust in God, and in a responsible and loving way, we can find a meaning both in our own and other's lives. This is also the case in situations that push us to our limits, as when we come face to face with a life-threatening illness.

The Bible and Christian tradition offer many stories of people who have been healed through divine intervention. But there are also stories of people affected by serious illnesses, accidents or losses who still find a way to live on. This can also be seen as a work of God. These are stories of how people have found not only a way of continuing to live, but also of living a life full of meaning and importance.

The Example of the Gospel

At the heart of a Christian view of humanity are both the experiences that we as Christians share with all human beings and the texts given to us in the Bible. These stories contain a dynamism that, even today, functions to help us interpret life. The stories must be re-interpreted in every era, and also relate to our experiences, for example, of HIV.

The central stories are naturally those about Jesus. In Jesus Christ, God shows, in a unique and eternally unsurpassable way, his love for all people and calls upon us to follow his lead. The ultimate confirmation of the value of human life is the Gospel story of how God himself was born in human form in Jesus. In this story, our own experience as people is mirrored, and God invites us to make the story of Jesus our own by following him on the path that leads through death to life.

There are, of course, no stories about HIV in the Bible. The closest we get are the stories about leprosy, for example, how Jesus cures ten lepers (Luke 17:11–19). Throughout the ages, leprosy has been a marginalized and stigmatized disease, just like HIV in our time. People saw those affected as unclean and banished them from social communion. The Bible shows how Jesus treats these people who are suffering and marginalized. However, there is a risk in reading the Gospels' stories of miraculous healing as if they were essentially about the disease. The Gospels are not primarily about how a person can be freed from disease, but rather who Jesus is and what God's will is with regard to human life. We discover the deeper contexts in our lives when we learn to look beyond the obvious.

In the Gospel of John, chapter 9, we find a story that is unusual in that Jesus comments on the condition with which he is faced and rejects the interpretation that everyone around him makes. His words help us not only to understand the concrete situation in the story, but also our own attitudes to illness and disability. The story starts with Jesus meeting a man who has been blind since birth.

"Rabbi, who sinned, this man or his parents, that he was born blind?" Jesus answers, "Neither this man nor his parents sinned; he was born blind so that God's works might be revealed in him." He spreads a paste of mud and saliva over the blind man's eyes and sends him off to wash in the pool of Siloam. The man returns from the pool able to see—and immediately comes into conflict with the religious leaders, who want to cast Jesus in an unfavorable light.

Speaking of Jesus, they say, "We know that this man is a sinner." The cured man answers, "I do not know whether he is a sinner. One thing I do know, that though I was blind, now I see." Later, he meets Jesus but without recognizing him—after all, he has never actually seen him. Jesus asks him, "Do you believe in the Son of Man?" and he answers, "And who is he, sir? Tell me, so that I may believe in him." When Jesus says to him "You have seen him, and the one speaking with you is he," the man declares his faith and falls at the feet of Jesus, who says, "I came into this world for judgment so that those who do not see may see, and those who do see may become blind."

The striking thing about this story is how Jesus rejects the assumption of his time that illness and disability are a direct consequence of someone's sin. He turns the perspective on its head. Instead, he gives meaning to the man's situation. Blindness and clarity of sight switch places: the blind man, who through his disability, was marginalized and so seen as a sinner, is freed from his marginalization and becomes the one who, through his faith, sees clearly. Those who see themselves as sighted are portrayed as blind inasmuch as they fail to understand who Jesus is, despite seeing him there in front of them. The experience of the formerly blind man is contrasted with the false sense of security of the Pharisees. As subject, his humanity restored, the congenitally blind man is even able to challenge the religious leaders of his time.

We who read the text are offered a choice between identifying with the blind man or with the Pharisees. A false sense of security can, unfortunately, appears to be an all too familiar attitude, not least in the materially secure existence that many people enjoy in a country such as Sweden.

But a crisis can become a turning point that allows us to discover life's real values.

The Gospel stories seek to help us find a deeper meaning in our lives. Illness and disability can become visible reminders that we are all essentially dependent on each other and the grace of God. Vulnerability in life is something that we all share, and once we realize that, we are already on the path towards a good life, full of empathy.

Ethical Points of Departure

HIV brings up fundamental questions about how we as people behave towards each other. HIV is sometimes referred to as "the great revealer" that forces us to talk about human behavior and attitudes that we neither want nor dare to speak about.

We see these as questions of ethics. Like life itself, an ethical discussion cannot be stated as a simple theoretical formula nor can it be reduced to a set of principles. Stories and examples are keys when it comes to understanding the morally relevant aspects of different situations. The tangibility of the stories can give substance and clarity to the principles. In Christian ethics, this is particularly true as regards the Gospel stories about Jesus—both what he said and what he did.

In the previous section, we gave an example of how the Bible can be used when reflecting on ethical issues. However, the Bible is not the only point of departure for Christian ethics. Like everyone else, we as Christians are required by Creation itself to be ethical in our relations with our fellow human beings. Creation is set up in such a way that we are dependent on each other. This comes into sharp focus at certain stages of our lives: we are utterly dependent when we are born, but also when we are very sick. Each and every one of us has a responsibility to meet the needs of other people when it is possible for us to do so. We may do this in our families, at work and in our local communities, but our responsibility for each other is not limited to the people who belong to the same group as we do: it applies to everyone, regardless of where we may happen to find ourselves.

When faced with other people's needs, it is often perfectly clear how we can help to make sure they are met. For instance, we do not need any biblical revelations to understand that a small child needs to be cared for. God created us with common sense and a conscience that we can use to understand how we should behave in different situations. We have a responsibility to make use of this gift to the best of our ability. This means that ethics is, to a large extent, rooted in Creation.

Ethics cannot be reduced to individual principles, but such principles can still assist us in clarifying our ethical arguments. Starting from the Bible and Creation, we can justify two important points of departure: the principle of human value and the concept of stewardship.

Both negative and positive duties follow from the *principle of human value*. The negative duties set the limits for how we can treat other people. They state what we may not do and express a respect for the integrity of the individual. For example, none of us has the right to exploit other people for our own purposes; we should always see our relationships with other as ends and not means. The negative duties also require that we refrain from actions that can hurt or offend other people.

The positive duties, on the other hand, require us to act in the interests of other people. This means that we are obliged to actively protect the rights and well-being of others. We also have to work for the fair distribution of the planet's resources and for equality between people. As such, the principle of human value places obligations on us concerning justice and solidarity, key elements of any ethic that seeks to safeguard values such as love, respect and reciprocity.

The *concept of stewardship* is also bound up with the view of the world as God's Creation. God has entrusted us with the resources of Creation, so that we may use them in the service of others. Created in God's image, we, as humans, are able to understand how various things relate, and human ingenuity has made it possible for us to make the most of the resources of Creation. From an ethical perspective, we can highlight two central aspects of the concept of stewardship. One relates to using the resources of Creation in order to improve human welfare and combat suffering and need, and the other relates to caring for and defending Creation, with respect for its integral value and with regard to the needs of future generations.

Scientific achievements have radically improved our ability to make use of the resources of Creation. Our lives have been made easier in so many ways through technical progress, and medical science has made it possible to conquer many illnesses. God, who is love and goodness, wants the resources of Creation to be used with responsibility and for the common good. Within The concept of stewardship, is predicated on that we, as humans, have been given freedom, at the same time as it is expected of us that we will remain faithful to the will of God.

Neither the principle of human value nor the concept of stewardship is exclusive to a Christian ethic. For instance, the idea that all people are equal lies at the heart of universally recognized human rights, and the concept of stewardship is brought into focus in the global debate on distribution issues, environmental destruction and the exploitation of non-renewable natural resources.

The principle of human value and the concept of stewardship are important points of departure as we seek a loving and responsible approach to HIV. According to the principle of human value, everyone affected has the right to receive care, loving support and medical help. This is also true for those children whose parents have died of AIDS or who are far too sick to be able to take care of them. Respect for the value of human life also obliges each and every one of us to behave responsibly in order to prevent the spread of HIV.

The concept of stewardship can motivate us to exploit the potential of science and make major investments in research to develop medication that prevents the progress of the disease, relieves the symptoms and hopefully, in the long term, provides a permanent cure.

It has already been established that the destructive effects of HIV and poverty are mutually reinforcing, and that this especially affects women. The HIV epidemic strengthens the arguments for fighting poverty that follow from both the principle of human value and the concept of stewardship. Among other things, it is a question of, in various ways, giving everyone infected with HIV access to the medication that is currently only available to those who can pay.

Working against HIV requires the commitment of enormous resources, which clearly has to be carried out at the societal level and globally. Information initiatives are one area that requires massive investment. At the same time, it is important to realize that we as individuals must also act responsibly, and that this cannot be delegated to someone else. Every one is responsible for their sexual relations and for getting tested if they suspect they may be infected. However, we are also obliged, in our own relations, to defend everyone's value and dignity, and to combat all discrimination in the contexts in which we move.

Respect for human life demands that no vulnerable person be discriminated against. It also means that no one can primarily see themselves or any fellow human being as a victim of circumstances beyond our control, or as an object of other peoples' benevolence. Respect for the value of every person requires us to see each other as the responsible subjects of our own lives.

From the Gospel stories about Jesus, we can discern the attitudes that should inform our relations, and that these attitudes should apply to everyone, even vulnerable persons. We need to show love, empathy, care, respect and fairness. In our shared aim of combating HIV we, as good stewards, must also efficiently exploit the resources at our disposal.

HIV in Churches' Pastoral Care

People affected by HIV are a challenge for the pastoral care of churches. HIV touches on our innermost integrity, not least because it is a sexually-transmitted disease. HIV engenders strong feelings of shame and guilt, both in relation to other people and in relation to a person's own situation. This is dealt with in different ways in different cultures. Reactions of repression, denial and silence are common. Fear of the reactions they expect makes people keep quiet instead of opening up for the conversations that can be the start of a positive development.

In pastoral care there is an atmosphere of security, which means that we dare to tell more than we have before—even about matters that we have kept secret, even from ourselves.

Dealing with guilt and dealing with shame are two separate processes that should not be conflated. The root of our guilt is concrete actions, or neglecting to act the way we think we ought to have. A healthy sense of guilt can most easily be described as regret or a bad conscience.

Many of those who receive an HIV diagnosis feel that they have brought it on themselves. This feeling seems to arise, no matter how a person becomes infected. In this context, no one can avoid dealing with the issue of responsibility. Coming to terms with what has happened, who or what is responsible and how it occurred can be a long process. Part of this process involves differentiating between what is real, "healthy" guilt and what is guilt about something for which the individual is not actually responsible.

To take responsibility for what you have done or omitted to do, to acknowledge and to regret is the path to release: that is how the guilt can be dealt with, forgiven and reconciled. Pastoral care can highlight the opportunity for openness, and hopefully also for reconciliation and forgiveness, in relation to other people. But in pastoral care the question of guilt and reconciliation are also related to God. Through Jesus Christ, we have the promise of redemption for all guilt. God's forgiveness is already there for us, ready to be given to those who ask for it. In individual pastoral care and in divine services, churches have a duty to convey this forgiveness.

When it comes to HIV, shame is often a major problem. We can cause each other pain by sending out the message of shame to each other. However, the message only gains a foothold when the shame has an ally in our own wounded inner self. Then the shame can prevent us from reacting with healthy anger towards those people who lack respect for us.

The unhealthy shame comes from how we perceive ourselves. It has its roots in our self-image, which has been created through the experiences that life has given us. A person who has been badly treated from the start, or who has been bombarded with messages that strengthen their sense of inferiority, finds it easy to feel like a worthless failure. To then be infected with HIV creates a whole new level of shame, both from the outside and the inside. It can be difficult to differentiate between the feelings that arise out of unhealthy and healthy shame. Here we often need help from outside, from people who are experts at seeing and understanding the difference. It is a frightening and new experience to act as if the shame did not exist: to dare to say no, to stand up for our own needs or to set boundaries when others lay on us a responsibility that is not ours. It is difficult, but every time we succeed in overcoming the shame, we feel its power fade.

Having the courage to tell other people that one is infected with HIV is an effective way of overcoming the shame. The pastoral caregiver can encourage this, and can be an important ally for those who feel that they are standing alone against the entire world.

The shame cannot be removed through forgiveness. On the contrary, it is disastrous when we ask for forgiveness for something that is not our responsibility. That simply deepens the shame. In this situation, there is a need for understanding, insight, and rehabilitation—perhaps during many conversations with a gentle, empathetic and understanding spiritual caretaker, someone who takes care of us and mourns with us as the truth emerges.

Talking with other people in groups can also be a way of rectifying a destructive self-image. Honest and open exchanges with others who are wrestling with the same issues are one of the very best ways of reducing the shame. That which has been wounded in relationships needs new relationships in order to heal. New accepting and loving relationships can lessen and eliminate the shame that has built up through early destructive relationships.

CONCLUSIONS AND RECOMMENDATIONS

> I don't want my church to say, "I can help you to die," but "Let me help you to live!"
>
> —Japé Heath
> South Africa
> priest and member of ANERELA+

Conclusions

Dealing with HIV reveals our deepest attitudes to the value and dignity of people and our fear of the unknown, not least our own mortality. Whether or not we are infected with HIV, we are forced to face up to the disease and to each other. Together, we will determine whether HIV spreads any further.

It is universally the case that HIV confronts us with questions of human dignity and of how we view humanity. The extent of the epidemic varies in different parts of the world, but the same questions of value arise everywhere: In Southern Africa, where the problems are numerically greatest, in Eastern Europe or Central and South East Asia, where the number of new cases is worryingly high—and in Sweden, despite worrying tendencies to trivialize the problem because of its relatively small scale.

The issue of HIV raises questions as to how we perceive other people and how we respect their inherent human dignity. The first and most obvious aspect of this, and the one thus far to receive most attention, deals with halting the spread of the epidemic and preventing people from dying of AIDS. Respect for the life of each individual requires that we focus on this. Considering the fact that it has long been known just how serious the

A Pastoral Letter from the Bishops of the Church of Sweden

situation is, it is practically incomprehensible that the global fight against HIV is not more extensive.

The second aspect has so far not received adequate attention. Insufficient resources are being put into breaking the "culture of silence" that surrounds HIV. For the person infected and for his or her family, the silence can be just as difficult to deal with as the disease itself. A global strategy for the value-related issues surrounding HIV is just as necessary as the global strategy in the epidemiological field.

In both these respects, churches have a key role to play in maintaining respect for the value of human life. A responsible and loving attitude in dealing with HIV requires that the epidemic and the risk of infection are taken extremely seriously, and that churches work together with other players to combat the spread of infection. Secondly, it also requires that those already infected be taken seriously. Dignity lies at the heart of all care and treatment. Dignity is necessary in all human contexts, not only in healthcare but also throughout society, including in churches and parishes. Churches should focus particularly on their vital role when it comes to value-related issues surrounding HIV. Churches, organizations and agencies should be encouraged to work in close partnership, so that the resources of the churches can be put to full use.

In the history of the Church of Sweden, it should be remembered that we showed solidarity with the people of Southern Africa in their fight against apartheid. Today, we have to show the same solidarity—with them, with each other and with everyone—in the fight against HIV. In both cases, it is a matter of standing up for the inviolable value of human life. HIV is an issue of life and death in many more respects than just expected lifespan. The question is what we all have to look forward to in our lives: love, empathy and dignity or shame, isolation and humiliation?

On such issues, all the world's churches have an answer, a greeting to every person from God who is the God of life. That message is in every sense a promise of life.

As churches, we must turn away from shaming persons who are infected with HIV. In individual pastoral care, churches' workers meet people who are infected with HIV or are concerned about HIV. Our task as churches and as Christians is to act as beacons of life, hope and meaning even in difficult situations. Being diagnosed with HIV should not be trivialized, but after the severe reactions that such a diagnosis can naturally cause, it is necessary to find a constructive approach to a new situation in life. In offering pastoral care, it is essential to maintain respect for the value of each person, and to strengthen each person's will to live in responsible and loving relationships. Those who already feel powerless, valueless and marginalized need more empathetic support to realize their opportunities and defend their human and moral integrity.

Those who regularly provide pastoral care to people should have sufficient knowledge about HIV not to be frightened of meeting infected people and their families. We in the churches should strive to express ourselves clearly on the issue of HIV and sexual relations, within pastoral care and in education and preaching. The silence that arises out of modesty must be broken if the spread of HIV is to be halted, and it is our duty to remind people just how vital it is to use condoms.

However, the importance of expressing ourselves clearly relates not only to concrete issues such as condom use or the promotion of other methods of prevention. We also need to speak positively and realistically about human sexuality, and we need to bring up fundamental, but often ignored, questions of people's ability to retain their sexual integrity. This applies not least to issues surrounding the sexual rights of women. Destructive social patterns must be challenged, even when they are part of a long tradition.

Churches are able, in various ways, to get involved in the care and treatment of HIV-infected and AIDS patients. In many countries, churches and religious organizations are by far the largest players in the healthcare sector, alongside national health services. Medication is a reality of life for the HIV-infected, and those living with HIV are, in many ways, on their own in their difficult situation. In this context, churches can provide support for the infected and his or her family.

Churches around the world have a key role to play in responding to HIV, but they have not always fully realized just how important their role is, both in terms of speaking out about the spread of infection and prevention and in terms of the underlying value-related issues. Very few players in civil society have such a great overall reach. In some countries, churches are the only movements operating from the suburbs of the cities to the most remote rural villages. Religious leaders, churches and faith-based organizations are, therefore, close to the most vulnerable groups and can promote prevention, care and treatment.

The Church of Sweden has a presence throughout the country, and its parishes reach not least a large proportion of young people. This gives the

A Pastoral Letter from the Bishops of the Church of Sweden

Church of Sweden opportunities to help young people gain a good understanding of what the disease means and how they can protect themselves. It also enables the Church of Sweden to take young peoples' insights and experiences into account and incorporate them into the ongoing work on issues of human dignity, determination and justice.

Added to this is the extraordinarily important role that the Church can play in the matter of shaping opinion and work on underlying values. This is true locally, nationally and globally. Churches must actively protest against active recruitment of medical staff by rich Western countries that leaves low-income countries stripped of valuable expertise. Churches must work to influence the pharmaceutical companies, so that they do not profit from the situation of poor people.

The role of churches in combating HIV is primarily to resist discrimination and stand up for people's rights and value in every way possible. We would urge all church workers and members, in conjunction with the annual World AIDS Day on 1 December, to make churches a prominent and committed force in society's manifestation against HIV, and also to raise the issues surrounding HIV prominently and forcefully in the heart of the parish. Naturally the HIV work must continue all year round, but World AIDS Day offers an opportunity to highlight the issues raised by HIV.

The Church of Sweden, together with other churches, must stand up for every person's right to care and treatment. In this context, no person or country should be seen chiefly in the light of their shortcomings, but in the light of their potential. HIV makes it possible and necessary for us to appreciate the equal value of everyone and everyone's shared vulnerability. This is the empathetic path that God himself showed by making Jesus Christ human for our sake.

Recommendations

Based on the points above, the Bishops of the Church of Sweden direct the following recommendations

To Swedish agencies and political decision-making bodies:

- that they increase initiatives to combat all tendencies towards discrimination on the grounds of HIV
- that they put more resources into HIV information for preventive purposes, particularly among young people

- that they increase international aid to projects aimed at protecting and strengthening the sexual and reproductive health and rights of everyone.

To UNAIDS and other international organizations tackling HIV issues:

- that they work with NGOs to develop a global strategy regarding value-related issues surrounding HIV.

To those responsible for healthcare resources in their country:

- that they strive to treat every patient well and with dignity in meeting their medical, social and spiritual needs
- that they refrain from actively recruiting medical staff and thereby contributing to the draining of healthcare systems in countries with widespread HIV infection.

To patent-holders and decision-makers in the pharmaceutical industry:

- that they honor their human responsibilities and use their resources in ways that benefits humanity
- that they increase initiatives to develop medication suitable for children
- that they respect the World Trade Organization's TRIPS Agreement and refrain from challenging and fighting poor countries' legal right to increase access to medication through their own production or through import of generic drugs
- that they adjust the pricing of their products in relation to what is reasonable considering the needs and resources of different countries.

To all parishes and workers in the churches:

- that they seek to increase their knowledge of the issues surrounding HIV
- that they make the most of their opportunities to influence young people and make them aware of the risk of HIV
- that they strive to make the parish a safe and trustworthy meeting place where everyone can feel welcome, important and valued.

To us church leaders around the world:

- that we all, in our own contexts, contribute to an increased competency in and theological reflection on HIV-related issues

A Pastoral Letter from the Bishops of the Church of Sweden

- that we work to increase knowledge about HIV and HIV prevention in our churches and set a good example by starting to talk about HIV ourselves
- that we, to save human lives, recommend that people use condoms
- that we develop pastoral expertise in our churches on the issues surrounding HIV
- that we stand up for the value of every human being, defend vulnerable groups and, in every way possible, combat discrimination.

Resources

ANERELA+
African Network of Religious Leaders Living with or Personally Affected by HIV & AIDS

    Address: 5th Floor JCC House, 27 Owl Street, Milpark, Johannesburg 2006, South Africa
    Phone: +27 11 482 9101
    Website: www.anerela.org
    E-mail: info@anerela.org

The Church of Sweden

    Postal address: SE-751 70 Uppsala, Sweden
    Visiting address: Sysslomansgatan 4, Uppsala, Sweden
    Phone: +46 (0)18-16 96 00
    Website: www.svenskakyrkan.se
    E-mail: info@svenskakyrkan.se

CDC
Centers for Disease Control and Prevention

    Programme within U.S. Department of Health & Human Services.
    Website: http://www.cdc.gov/hiv/

Circle of Concerned African Women Theologians

    The Circle is the space for women from Africa to do communal theology, to undertake research and publish theological literature written by African women with special focus on religion and culture.
    Website: http://www.thecirclecawt.org/

Resources

EAA
Ecumenical Advocacy Alliance

Ecumenical network for international cooperation in advocacy on HIV-related issues.
Website: www.e-alliance.ch

EHAIA
The Ecumenical Response to HIV/AIDS in Africa

Programme within the World Council of Churches which gives churches in Africa access to information, training, networking and support in their work with HIV in their local communities.
Website: www.wcc-coe.org/wcc/what/mission/ehaia-e.html

HAI
Harvard School of Public Health AIDS Initiative

Website promoting research, education and leadership to end the AIDS epidemic.
Website: http://www.hsph.harvard.edu/hai/

HIV InSite

Information on HIV and AIDS treatment, prevention, and policy from the University of California San Francisco
Website: http://hivinsite.ucsf.edu/

IAS
International AIDS Society

International organisation for researchers working on HIV and AIDS. IAS also organises scientific conferences and congresses.
Website: www.ias.se

INERELA+
International Network of Religious Leaders Living with or Personally Affected by HIV & AIDS

Address: 5th Floor JCC House, 27 Owl Street, Milpark, Johannesburg 2006, South Africa
Phone: +27 11 482 9101
Website: www.inerela.org

Resources

Swedish Institute for Infectious Disease Control

> Central administrative agency responsible for monitoring the epidemiological situation regarding infectious diseases among the population and with promoting protection against such diseases.
> Website: www.smittskyddsinstitutet.se

UNAIDS
The Joint United Nations Programme on HIV/AIDS

> The website posts important documents and statistics about HIV.
> Website: www.unaids.org

WHO
World Health Organization

> Aims to achieve the best possible health for people everywhere. WHO leads and coordinates health work within the UN.
> Website: www.who.int/hiv/en/

Bibliography

"2007 AIDS epidemic update." *UNAIDS*. Online: http://www.unaids.org/en/Knowledge Centre/HIVData/EpiUpdate/EpiUpdArchive/2007/.

Ackermann, Denise. "Tamar's Cry: Re-Reading an Ancient Text in the Midst of an HIV and AIDS Pandemic." In *Grant Me Justice: HIV/AIDS & Gender Readings of the Bible*, edited by Musa W. Dube, and Musimbi R.A. Kanyoro, 27–59. Maryknoll, N.Y.: Orbis Books, 2004.

———. "HIV- and AIDS-related stigma: implications for theological education, research, communication and community stigma: implication for the theological agenda." In *A Report of a Theological Workshop Focusing on HIV- and AIDS-related Stigma*, 46–50. Geneva: UNAIDS, 2005.

A Report of a Theological Workshop Focusing on HIV and AIDS-related Stigma. Geneva: UNAIDS, 2005.

Auvert, B. et al. "Randomised, controlled intervention trial of male circumcision for reduction of HIV infection risk: the ANRS 1265 Trial." *PLos Med.* 2 (11) e298 (2005).

Bernardin, Joseph. *A Moral Vision for America*. Washington, D.C.: Georgetown University Press, 1998.

———. *Consistent Ethic of Life*. Kansas City: Sheed & Ward, 1988.

Bonaseo, Bernardino M., O.F.M. *Man and His Approach to God in John Duns Scotus*. Lanham, Md.: University Press of America, 1983.

Bongmba, Elias K. *Facing a Pandemic: The African Church and the Crisis of HIV/AIDS*. Waco: Baylor University Press, 2007.

Boniface-Male, Anastasia. "Allow Me to Cry Out: Reading of Mathew 15:21–28 in the Context of HIV/AIDS in Tanzania." In *Grant Me Justice: HIV/AIDS & Gender Readings of the Bible*, edited by Musa W. Dube, and Musimbi R.A. Kanyoro, 169–85. Maryknoll, N.Y.: Orbis Books, 2004.

Brown, Raymond E. *The Gospel According to John (i–xii)*. Garden City, N.Y.: Doubleday & Company, 1966.

Brownmiller, Susan. *Against our Will: Men Women and Rape*. New York: Ballantine Books, 1993.

Brueggemann, Walter. "The Costly Loss of Lament." *Journal for the Study of the Old Testament* vol. 36 (1986).

Cahill, Lisa Sowle. "The Atonement Paradigm." *Theological Studies* vol. 68, no. 2 (June 2007) 418–32.

"Called to be the One Church. *World Council of Churches.* "The Ninth Assembly of the World Council of Churches. Online: http://www.oikoumene.org/en/resources/documents/assembly/porto-alegre-2006/1-statements-documents-adopted/

Bibliography

christian-unity-and-message-to-the-churches/called-to-be-the-one-church-as-adopted.html.
Called to Compassion and Responsibility. National Conference of Catholic Bishops. Washington: USCC Office of Publishing Services, 1990.
Carpenter, Stephen. "What perceived benefits do HIV positive patients on antiretroviral therapy derive from participation in a local church? The experience of patients at Valley Trust ARV centre." Masters Thesis, University of KwaZulu-Natal, 2007.
Chauke, Elisinah. "Theological Challenges and Ecclesiological Responses to Women Experiencing HIV & AIDS: A South Eastern Zimbabwe Context." In *African Women, Religion, and Health: Essays in the Honor of Mercy Amba Ewudwiza Oduyoye*, edited by Isabel Apawo Phiri, and Sarojini Nadar, 128–48. Maryknoll, N.Y.: Orbis Books, 2006.
Chitando, Ezra. *Living with Hope. African Churches and HIV/AIDS 1.* Geneva: WCC Publications, 2007.
———. *Acting in Hope. African Churches and HIV/AIDS 2.* Geneva: WCC Publications, 2007.
Cimperman, Maria. *When God's People have HIV/AIDS. An Approach to Ethics.* Maryknoll, N.Y.: Orbis Books, 2005.
Collins, Joseph, and Bill Rau, *AIDS in the Context of Development.* UNRISD Programme on Social Policy and Development Paper Number 4, UNRISD. Geneva: United Nations Research Institute for Social Development, December 2000.
"Compassion, Conversion, Care: Responding as churches to the HIV/AIDS pandemic. An Action Plan of the Lutheran World Federation." Geneva, 2002. Online: http://www.lutheranworld.org/LWF_Documents/HIVAIDS-Action-plan.pdf.
Crossan, John Dominic. *Jesus: A Revolutionary Biography.* New York: HarperSanFrancisco, 1994.
Daly, Mary. *Beyond God the Father: Toward a Philosophy of Women's Liberation.* Boston: Beacon Press, 1985.
"Debt-for-AIDS Swaps," *UNAIDS.* Online: http://www.unaids.org/en/default.asp, then use search for title.
Dewey, Arthur J. *The Word in Time.* Rev. ed. New Berlin, Wis.: Liturgical Publications, 1990.
———. "Can We Let Jesus Die." In *The Once & Future Faith*, edited by Robert W. Funk, et al., 135–59. Santa Rosa, Polebridge Press, 2001.
———. "The Truth That Is In Jesus." *The Fourth R* (July–August 2003) 7–11.
Dube, Musa W. "Preaching to the Converted: Unsettling the Christian Church." *Ministerial Formation* 93 (2001) 38–50.
———. "Theological Challenges: Proclaiming the Fullness of Life in the HIV/AIDS and Global Economic Era." *International Review of Mission* vol. XCI, no. 363 (2002) 523–49.
———. *Africa Praying: A Handbook on HIV/AIDS Sensitive Sermons Guidelines and Liturgy.* Geneva: WCC, 2003.
———. *HIV/AIDS and the Curriculum: Methods of Integrating HIV/AIDS in Theological Programs.* Geneva: WCC, 2003.
———. "Twenty-Two Years of Bleeding and Still the Princess Sings!" In *Grant Me Justice: HIV/AIDS & Gender Readings of the Bible*, edited by Musa W. Dube, and Musimbi R.A. Kanyoro, 186–200. Maryknoll, N.Y.: Orbis Books, 2004.

Bibliography

———. "Theological Education: HIV/AIDS and Other Challenges in the New Mellennium," In *Theological Education in Contemporary Africa*, edited by Grant LeMarquand, and Joseph D. Galgalo, 105–30. Eldoret: A Zapf Chancery, 2004.
Dube, Musa W., and Musimbi Kanyoro. *Grant Me Justice: HIV/AIDS & Gender Readings of the Bible*. Maryknoll, N.Y.: Orbis Books, 2004.
Dulles, Avery. *Models of the Church*. Expanded Edition. New York, N.Y.: Doubleday, 1987 (1974).
Dych, William. *Karl Rahner*. Collegeville: The Liturgical Press, 1992.
Elliott, John H. "Patronage and Clientism in Early Christian Society," *Forum* vol. 3, no. 4 (December 1987).
Epstein, Helen. *The Invisible Cure: Africa, the West, and the fight against AIDS*. New York: Farrar, Straus and Giroux, 2007.
Erikson, Erik. *Childhood and Society*. New York, London: Norton, 1963.
———. *Identity and the Life Cycle*. New York, London: Norton, 1980.
"Facing AIDS: Education in the Context of Vulnerability HIV/AIDS." *World Council of Churches*. Online: http://www.wcc-coe.org/wcc/what/mission/facing2.html.
Faley, Roland J. "Leviticus." In *The New Jerome Biblical Commentary*, edited by Raymond Brown et al., 69–70. Englewood Cliffs: Prentice Hall, 1990.
"'Forgive and Forget' Won't Fix Third World Debt," *Worldwatch Institute*. Online: http://www.worldwatch.org/press/news/2001/04/261.
Garcia-Moreno, Claudia et al. "Violence against Women." *Science*, vol. 310 no. 5752 (2005), 1282–83.
Gilligan, Carol. *In a Different Voice: Psychological Theory and Women's Development*. Cambridge: Harvard University Press, 1982.
Grace, Care and Justice, A handbook for HIV and AIDS work. Geneva: Lutheran World Federation, 2007.
Gutierrez, Gustavo. *On Job*. Maryknoll, N.Y.: Orbis Books, 1987.
Harrington, Daniel. *Why Do We Suffer?* Franklin, Wis.: Sheed & Ward, 2000.
Hartung, William D., and Frida Berrigan. "Militarization of U.S. African Policy, 2000 to 2005." *World Policy Institute* Online: http://www.worldpolicy.org/projects/arms/reports.html.
Heath, Johannes Petrus. "HIV- and AIDS-related Stigma: Living With the Experience." In *A Report of a Theological Workshop Focusing on HIV and AIDS-related Stigma*, 27–31. Geneva: UNAIDS, 2005.
Hill, Brennan. *Jesus, the Christ*. New ed. Mystic, Conn: Twenty-Third Publications, 2004.
Himes, Kenneth R. *Modern Catholic Social Teaching*. Washington, D.C.: Georgetown University Press, 2005.
Hooks, Bell. *Black Looks: Race Representation*. Boston: South End, 1992.
"Intensifying HIV prevention: a UNAIDS policy position paper." Geneva: UNAIDS, August 2005. Online: http://data.unaids.org/publications/irc-pub06/jc1165-intensif_hiv-newstyle_en.pdf.
Irwin, Alexander et al. *Global AIDS: Myths and Facts: tools for fighting the AIDS pandemic*. Cambridge, Mass.: South End Press, 2003.
Isaak, Paul John. "The Compassionate God—John 11." In *God Breaks the Silence: In Preaching in Times of AIDS*, 135–37. Wuppertal: UEM, 2005.
Jewkes, Rachel. 2005. "Non-consensual sex among South African youth: Prevalence of coerced sex and discourses of control and desire." *Journal of Infectious Diseases* 15 189:10 (2004), 1785–92.

Bibliography

John XXIII. "Peace on Earth." In *The Gospel of Peace and Justice*, edited by Joseph Gremillion. Maryknoll, N.Y.: Orbis Books, 1976.

John Paul II. *On Social Concern*. Washington, D.C.: USCC Office of Publishing Services, 1987.

———. *The Gospel of Life*. Boston: Pauline Books & Media, 1995.

Kammer, Fred. *Doing Faithjustice*. Mahwah, N.J.: Paulist Press, 1991.

Kanyoro, Musimbi. "Preface: Breaking the Silence on HIV & AIDS: The Lament of Women of Africa." In *African women, HIV/ AIDS, and Faith Communities*, edited by Isabel Apawo Phiri et al., xi–xii. Pietermaritzburg: Cluster Publications, 2003.

Kharises, Julieth. "Effective pastoral care and counselling to parishioners contracted with HIV/AIDS: Women in the ELCRN." Masters Thesis, University of KwaZulu-Natal, 2000.

Kobia, Samuel. "Epiphany 2007 Message." *World Council of Churches*. Online: http://www.oikoumene.org/en/resources/documents/general-secretary/messages-and-letters/09-01-07-epiphany-letter.html.

Kolvenbach, Peter-Hans, S.J., "The Service of Faith and the Promotion of Justice in American Jesuit Higher Education," *Santa Clara University* Online: http://www.scu.edu/ignatiancenter/bannan/eventsandconferences/lectures/archives/kolvenbach.cfm.

LaCugna, Catherine. *God for Us*. New York: HarperSanFrancisco, 1991.

Lamptey Peter R. "Reducing heterosexual transmission of HIV in poor countries." In *BMJ* 324:7331 (January 26, 2002), 207–11. Online: http://www.bmj.com/cgi/content/full/324/7331/207.

Landman, Christina. "Spiritual Care-giving to Women Affected by HIV & AIDS." In *African women, HIV/ AIDS, and Faith Communities*, edited by Isabel Apawo Phiri et al., 189–208. Pietermaritzburg: Cluster Publications, 2003.

Linked for Life. African Jesuit AIDS Network. Nairobi: Paulines Publications Africa, 2007.

Maluleke, Tinyiko Sam. "Towards an HIV/AIDS-Sensitive Curriculum." In *HIV/AIDS and the Curriculum: Methods of Integrating HIV/AIDS in Theological Programs*, edited by Musa W. Dube, 60–78. Geneva: WCC Publications, 2003.

Meier, John P. "Jesus." In *New Jerome Biblical Commentary*, edited by Raymond Brown et al., 1318–28. Englewood Cliffs: Prentice Hall, 1990.

Messer, Donald. *Breaking the Conspiracy of Silence: Christian Churches and the Global AIDS Crisis*. Minneapolis: Fortress Press, 2004.

Moloney, Francis J. *The Gospel of John*. Collegeville: The Liturgical Press, 1998.

Mooney, Christopher, S.J. *Teilhard de Chardin and the Mystery of Christ*. New York: Harper & Row, 1966.

Morris, Martina. *Aids in Uganda: Analysis of the Social Dimensions of the Epidemic*. Kampala: Makerere University, 2000.

Morris, Martina, and Mirjam Kretzschmar. "A Microsimulation Study of the Effect of Concurrent Partnerships on the Spread of HIV in Uganda." *Mathematical Population Studies* 8(2) (2000), 109–33.

Moyo, Fulata L. "Navigating Experiences of Healing: A Narrative Theology of Eschatological Hope as Healing." In *African Women, Religion, and Health: Essays in the Honor of Mercy Amba Ewudwiza Oduyoye*, edited by Isabel Apawo Phiri, and Sarojini Nadar, 243–53. Maryknoll, N.Y.: Orbis Books, 2006.

Mull, Kenneth V., and Carolyn Sandquist Mull. "Biblical Leprosy: Is It Really?" *Bible Review* vol. 8 (April 1992).

Bibliography

Nouwen Henri, et al. *Compassion: A Reflection on the Christian Life.* New York: Image Books Doubleday, 1982.

"Nurturing Peace, Overcoming Violence." *World Council of Churches.* Faith and Order Team, World Council of Churches. Online: http://www.oikoumene.org/en/resources/documents/wcc-commissions/faith-and-order-commission/viii-theological-reflection-on-peace/nurturing-peace-overcoming-violence-in-the-way-of-christ-for-the-sake-of-the-world.html.

"On the Situation in the Horn of Africa. *World Council of Churches.* "Executive Committee of the World Council of Churches. Online: http://www.oikumene.org/en/resources/document/executive-committee/geneva-march-2007/01-03-07-statement-on-the-situation-in-the-horn-of-africa.html.

Overberg, Kenneth R. S.J., *Ethics and AIDS: Compassion and Justice in Global Crisis.* Lanham, Md.: Rowman & Littlefield Publishers, 2006.

———. *Into the Abyss of Suffering.* Cincinnati: St. Anthony Messenger Press, 2003.

Paterson, Gillian. *Women in the Time of AIDS.* Maryknoll, N.Y.: Orbis Books, 1996.

Phiri, Isabel Apawo, et al. *African women, HIV/ AIDS, and Faith Communities.* Pietermaritzburg: Cluster Publications, 2003.

Phiri, Isabel Apawo, and Sarojini Nadar. "Introduction: Treading Softly but Firmly." In *African Women, Religion, and Health: Essays in the Honor of Mercy Amba Ewudwiza Oduyoye,* edited by Isabel Apawo Phiri, and Sarojini Nadar, 1–13. Maryknoll, N.Y.: Orbis Books, 2006.

Pilcher, Christopher D. et al. "Brief but efficient: acute HIV infection and the sexual transmission of HIV." *Journal of Infectious Diseases* 15 189:10 (2004), 1785–92.

Purvis, Sally B. "Compassion." In *Dictionary of Feminist Theologies,* edited by Letty Russell & J. Shannon Clackson, 51–52. Louisville: John Knox Press, 1996.

Rahner, Karl. "Thoughts on the Possibility of Belief Today." In Karl Rahner, *Theological Investigations,* vol. V. Baltimore: Helicon Press, 1966.

———. *Foundations of Christian Faith.* New York: The Seabury Press, 1978.

———. "Why Am I a Christian Today?" In *The Practice of Faith,* edited by Karl Lehmann, and Albert Raffelt. New York: The Crossroad Publishing Company, 1986.

Rehle, Thomas et al. 2007. "National HIV incidence measures—new insights into the South African epidemic." In *SAMJ,* vol. 97 no. 9 (2007) 194–99.

Report on the Global HIV/AIDS Epidemic. Geneva: UNAIDS, 2002.

Russell, Letty M. *The Church With AIDS: Renewal in the Midst of Crisis.* Louisville: WJKB, 1990.

———. "Re-Imagining the Bible in a Pandemic of HIV/AIDS." In *Grant Me Justice: HIV/ AIDS & Gender Readings of the Bible,* edited by Musa W. Dube, and Musimbi R.A. Kanyoro, 201–10. Maryknoll, N.Y.: Orbis Books, 2004.

Russell-Coons, Ron. "We have AIDS." In *The Church With AIDS: Renewal in the Midst of Crisis,* edited by Letty Russell, 35–55. Louisville: WJKB, 1990.

Schillebeeckx, Edward. *Jesus.* New York: The Seabury Press, 1979.

———. *Christ: The Experience of Jesus as Lord.* New York: The Seabury Press, 1980.

Schneiders, Sandra. *New Wineskins.* New York: Paulist, 1986.

Schoepf, Brooke Grundfest. "Health, Gender Relations, and Poverty in the AIDS Era." In *Courtyards, Markets, City Streets: Urban Women in Africa,* edited by Kathleen Sheldon. Boulder, Colo: Westview Press, 1996.

Bibliography

Scott, Christina. "'Alarming' HIV rise in young South African women." *Science and Development Network*. March 2005. Online: http://www.scidev.net/en/news/alarming-hiv-rise-in-young-south-african-women.html.

Simmermacher, Gunther. "The Body of Christ has Aids. Towards a new Aids theology." *The Southern Cross Editorial* (2003).

Skylstad, William. "Letter to President Bush: The G-8 Summit." *Origins* vol. 35, no. 8.

Smith, Ann, and Enda McDonagh, *The Reality of AIDS*. Maynooth, Ireland: Trocaire, Veritas, CAFOD, 2003.

Sniegocki, John. "The Social Ethics of Pope John Paul II." *Horizons* vol. 33, no. 1 (Spring 2006).

Sobrino, Jon. *Christology at the Crossroads*. Maryknoll, N.Y.: Orbis Books, 1978.

———. *Where Is God?* Maryknoll, N.Y.: Orbis Books, 2004.

"Statement on Latin America," *World Council of Churches*. The Ninth Assembly of the World Council of Churches, Online: http://www.oikoumene.org/en/resources/documents/assembly/porto-alegre-2006/1-statements-documents-adopted/international-affairs/report-from-the-public-issues-committee/latin-america.html.

Synod of Bishops, "Justice in the World." In *Gospel of Peace and Justice*, In *The Gospel of Peace and Justice*, edited by Joseph Gremillion. Maryknoll, N.Y.: Orbis Books, 1976.

Tambasco, Anthony J. *A Theology of Atonement and Paul's Vision of Christianity*. Collegeville: The Liturgical Press, 1991.

"The Swedish Institute for Infectious Disease Control" Online: www.smittskyddsinstitutet.se/statistik/hivinfektion.

"Towards a Policy on HIV/AIDS." *World Council of Churches*. Programme for Justice, Diakonia and Responsibility for Creation, World Council of Churches. Online: http://www.oikoumene.org/en/resources/documents/wcc-programmes/justice-diakonia-and-responsibility-for-creation/health-and-healing/hivaids/wcc-statements-and-studies/2006-towards-a-policy-on-hivaids.html.

Vatican II. "Church in the Modern World." In *Gospel of Peace and Justice*, edited by Joseph Gremillion. Maryknoll, N.Y.: Orbis Books, 1976.

Ward, Edwina. *A Theology of HIV & AIDS on Africa's East Coast*. Pietermaritzburg: Cluster Publications, 2008.

"What Does God Require of Us?" *World Council of Churches*. World Council of Churches. Online: http://www. oikoumene.org/en/resources/documents/wcc-programmes/public-witness-addressing-power-affirming-peace/economic-justice/trade/01-04-just-trade-declaration.html.

Wink, Walter. *Engaging the Powers*. Minneapolis: Fortress Press, 1992.

Winter, Michael. *The Atonement*. Collegeville: The Liturgical Press, 1995.

www.ingramcontent.com/pod-product-compliance
Lightning Source LLC
Chambersburg PA
CBHW070933160426
43193CB00011B/1672